VEGAN MEAL PREP AND PLANT-BASED DIET COOKBOOK FOR BEGINNERS

Vegan & Vegetarian Diet Book with High-Protein Meal Plans for Muscle Growth – Delicious & Easy Gluten-Free Recipes for a Healthy Lifestyle

Table of Contents

Introduction

Vegans do not consume animal fat or cholesterol, so they are less likely to develop cardiovascular disease (which is very common in meat consumers). Cardiovascular disease kills 1 million Americans annually.

Many people who follow the vegan diet report that their hair and nails are getting stronger and healthier, their allergies are gone, their acne and other skin problems are gone, their energy levels have increased.

In this exclusive guide I will cover everything you need to know about the Vegan diet and how to get started. Aside from being a nutritional beginner's guide, it serves as a cookbook with over 100 essential recipes and plant-based high protein recipes.

Veganism is not just a diet but also a lifestyle choice. A vegan diet can help with weight loss, reduce the risk of certain diseases, and improve your energy levels. If you want to increase your chances of sticking to this diet, concentrating on the food you consume should be your priority.

Meal prepping is essentially the practice of preparing wholesome meals, along with preparing certain components of the meals for the week ahead. In the last couple of years, this concept has steadily gained a lot of popularity. In this book, you'll find some amazing Vegan recipes that will get you started on your meal prep journey.

Once you start meal prepping, you can forget about takeout and fast food! You can start saving money, eating home-cooked meals, and improving your health. By using the different recipes given in this book, you can begin prepping meals like a pro. In today's world, it is quite easy to fall into the habit of eating fast food. Regardless of whether you are trying a plant-based diet or are weakened by choice, it can become a little challenging, since finding vegan options is not always easy. Rather than depending on restaurants or food bars for your vegan meals, start meal prepping today and get access to home-cooked ready to eat.

Are you ready to learn more about all this? If yes, then let us get started immediately.

Chapter 1: What Is Vegan?

Through eliminating animal products such as beef, fish, dairy products, milk, oil, jelly, lanolin, wool, fur, silk, suede and leather, veganism is the method of minimizing damage to all species. It's more than just a diet. It is a way of life that seeks to exclude animals by animal nutrition, clothes or other uses from any form of exploitation and cruelty.

Vegetarians do not consume meat or fish, but include other foods such as eggs and dairy products in their diet.

Vegan people have plenty to cook! I know when you start, there seems to be nothing to eat. Yet if you understand something, vegan food is fun, delicious, and nutritious. I don't feel like I'm missing anything.

Vegan diets consist only of vegetable-based foods, but vegans eat many of the same foods as non-vegans: pasta, rice, potatoes, salads, burgers, chips, tacos and even pizzas. Essentially, anything made from animal products can be vegan as well.

A diet based on vegetables is anything but animal products. Food groups consist of whole grains, fruits and vegetables, nuts, seeds and legumes.

Whole grain products include spaghetti, bread, rice, quinoa, beans, meal and other whole grain products. However, whole grain diets make up a large part of your diet and provide a great deal of your protein, fats, complex carbohydrates, vitamins, and minerals.

Plant: A large part of your diet is made up of vegetables and omnivores. These are low in calories but high in fiber, organic, phytochemical, and satisfy many nutritional requirements.

The only plants you can eat every day are dark green leafy greens. You should also think about eating as many different colors of vegetables as possible on a regular basis.

It is recommended that you eat at least one salad a day and add more vegetables to your daily diet by adding them to smoothies, soups, stews, and everything else.

Fruit: Several portions of fruit a day are a fantastic way to better meet your nutritional needs, particularly to improve the intake of antioxidants for disease. Fruit is rich in calories, minerals, vitamins and phytochemicals.

Refined fats from oils are not needed for optimal health, as the essential fats present in them are already available from the food sources of a healthy plant diet.

We will fulfill most of our essential fatty acid requirements by including avocados, olives, nuts and seeds in our diet while using other nutrients and fiber. The oil consumption should be kept to a minimum if a minimal amount of oil is perfect.

The veggie enthusiast diet is known for is medical benefits, and especially - weight loss. Various individuals have undergone the veggie lover diet for the only reason to get fit, and have predominant with respect to doing such. If that you're interested in finding a solid and secure eating routine for healthier and are considering the vegetarian diet, then you need to ask yourself: is it secure? Might it be astute? Is it possible?

In the event that you encounter the vegetarian diet in an honest, well-arranged manner, you may be sure that it's equally secure and strong. You need to ensure that you're ingesting a broad selection of nourishments always to ensure that you're accepting perfect sustenance - nevertheless hello, you need to get this done on any eating regime. If you somehow were able to drop back on eating veggie enthusiast low excellent nourishment all the time, your health would obviously endure.

Veggie lover low-quality nourishment comprises packaged crisps, chips that are hot, with no milk chocolate and parts of candies, alleged 'health bars' which are pressed with sugars and so on. Should you somehow be able to expend nourishments, as an instance, that all of the time and eat them rather than your proper suppers, you're damaging your body? Instead, you can choose to create your own vegetarian preparing strategies, by way of instance, without milk, low-sugar snacks, brownies, cakes, oat and nut cuts, so on., such as dates, dried organic goods, crisp all-natural goods, nuts, coconut oil, extra-virgin olive seeds, and oil. Experience your eating regimen in a judicious and continuous manner, and provide your body with the nutritional supplements that it requires.

Might it be astute?

In case you need to shed weight, the veggie lover diet is one of those good eating regimens which it is possible to adapt to perform as such. It's rash to choose a fad diet that's low in fat, saturated in leaves and supplements one feeling denied. It's possible to enjoy avocadoes, olive oil, seeds and nuts with this particular eating regimen - maybe not at all like most injury abstains from food now. You may likewise appreciate a range of gourmet, strong cooking so that you won't need to feel refused. By producing your own heavenly and strong veggie fan heating plans, you're guaranteeing you will stay happy and chemical with this eating regimen, instead of frustrated and grumpy.

So, if the veggie lover diet offers you a great deal of sound nutritional supplements, provides your body sufficient sound fats and does not leave you feeling denied, alright say it is wise or indiscreet to drift down this pathway? I'd say it is savvy.

Is it sensible?

There are some long drag veggie fans who've been on the vegetarian diet as long as they can recall or for quite a very long moment. These people are always lean and thin and possess a solid, shiny composition along with also a get-up-and-go that most are desirous of. Not at all like injury eats, this eating routine is reasonable. Why? You won't feel denied since there are a lot of yummy choices to consume. You're able to enjoy a broad range of beautiful veggie-lover heating programs or dinner programs, which can be anything but hard to find in books, on the internet, or by vegetarian formula electronic publications. The health care benefits of the eating regimen can permit you to understand it is well-worth neglecting meat and meat products. Several have completed as such and therefore are moving to do so now. Could this be you?

Weight loss on the vegetarian diet is sheltered, educated and economical. So perhaps it's now a chance to drop the entirety of your injury diet musings and thoughts, and select rather a solid, veggie enthusiast way of life which can leave your life components happy, strong and well-supported.

The talk of whether the vegetarian diet is unfortunate or sound is not new. The majority of people may say that an individual that embraces veganism will probably be inadequate in fundamental supplements found obviously in animal products, to be particular, animal-based protein. These individuals treasure the certainty that milk can keep their bones strong and red meat will provide standard protein to your own muscles.

Then again, there's a little minority of individuals (2 percent veggie lover and 5 percent vegetarian) who provide credit into the plant-based eating regimen relieving their real health problems, enabling them to get rid of overabundance weight, clearing their skin up and sensitivities, also providing them an astonishing pizzazz.

So, determined by those two contrasts in evaluations, how could one determine whether the veggie lover diet is undesirable or solid? Everything boils down to, not things 'conclusion,' nevertheless instead, on powerful actualities, evidence, contextual investigations and fair accounts of real people.

An honest vegetarian diet may be mind-blowing for your own wellbeing. Evidently, the puzzle is maintaining it corrected. An eating pattern of just veggie-lover treats, whilst vegetarian, wouldn't be strong by any stretch of the imagination. Sticking to some reasonable eating routine and ensuring to consume nourishments with some restraint is going to help you with being more valuable and becoming thinner. Really, even people that are as of today in a solid weight land will feel much better if their own body flushes the animal things out.

Benefits of a vegan diet and the human body was designed to be performed

The human body wasn't intended to consume meat and not milk, but rather for a plant amicable veggie enthusiast diet. We've got over 30 dissimilarities with carnivores, which can be likenesses we discuss with herbivores about our strategy. For example, our gut-associated tract is a very long plant encouraging you. A real flesh-eater includes a brief stomach associated tract and beef is completed in 3-7 hours. This will not allow parasites to bring forth. In individuals it takes three days to process beef, giving it ample moment for parasites to bring forth. That's a significant bit of the estimated 90 percent of people have parasites!

Anyway, we've got nails rather than pins, varied gut corrosiveness, spit, and our teeth arrangement is similar to herbivores and surely not a carnivore. It is in our impulses not to eat meat too. For example, on the off likelihood that you just saw a deceased bovine on the bud, you would not start salivating or will need to consume it like this. A real meat-eater would consume off. The major way you'd need it's if that you cooked it, in crops oils, and prepared it using herbs, etc. This is also since you've grown up eating beef so have been used to it. Be as it may, the body wasn't meant for meat, nevertheless instead a veggie fan diet.

Meat is full of saturated fats and less pristine as plants. Also, if your beef is not organic, grass-encouraged, and unfenced, you need to handle improvement hormones, anti-toxins, and steroids. All of that develops you and causes you to increasingly impervious to antimicrobials. Additionally, any uneasiness, also anxiety the monster underwent in its own life made artificial reactions within the body, by way of instance, enlarged levels of cortisol and adrenaline, which you have it, wind up in you. No major surprise such enormous numbers of people are mad and once we believe veggie fans, we believe smooth, relaxed people. Additionally, meat is indeed hard to process. Assimilation takes up the larger portion of your energy for the day. If that you're processing mangoes versus beef, that do you think is more faithfully on the human body and provides you more energy to do everything you need to do?

Additional dairy is extremely alarming. It is the absolute most noticeably dreadful everything being equivalent. We take milk, normally from an abused bovine who's given steroids, hormones, and antimicrobials, and cook it. Any nutritional supplements in the milk are presently gone, in fact, the milk is still acidic. We at the point brace the milk together with calcium and nutrients, however, it's not really the real article. At the stage when it pops up on your body it's acidic to the stage your body should use its magnesium and calcium save simply to kill the causticity. So's right, milk actually exhausts your assortment of calcium. You've lately been dissipated of possibly the most wonderful dream within recent memory. Additionally, milk is similarly full of malodorous fats also leaves you to put on fat efficiently. Think about what that milk has been intended for, baby dairy animals. That kid cow develops a lot of pounds in its first season only off this milk.

How it works

The vegan diet is a strict vegetarian diet. Vegan not only prohibits meat and fish, but also dairy products such as milk, eggs and gelatin, as well as animal foods such as honey.

Like all other types of eating, the same applies to vegan diets. The best combination of nutrients is a diverse selection of different foods.

Significant sources of non-vegan iron, calcium, iodine, vitamin D and B12 are animal foods such as meat, fish and dairy products. The following foods are therefore important for a healthy vegan diet: good sources of iron are green vegetables such as chard and spinach, legumes such as lentils and beans, and grain products such as oatmeal.

Among green vegetables and herbs such as broccoli, fennel, basil, and petroleum, essential calcium is extracted. Calcium is also found in nuts and seeds such as hazelnuts and sesame.

Iodine mainly provides sea-living food. With vegan diets, algae or iodized table salt works well.

In addition to animal products, in fermented products such as sauerkraut and beer, vitamin B12 is also found in trace components. For example, in mushrooms, vitamin D is found, but is also produced by the body itself.

There are no signs of lack shortages from vegan eating of varied and conscious food choices. Vegan diets often provide the body with much healthier vitamins and minerals as fresh fruits and vegetables substitute high-energy foods such as meat and sausages.

Vegan diet is an issue because food choices are one-sided and the opportunity for under-nutrition is too little awareness. Nutrients such as vitamin B12 are urgently required, especially during pregnancy and lactation and during childhood. Third, dietary supplements can be of help to your vegan diet.

Types of vegan diet

Ovo lacto vegetarians do not eat fish or meat. For example, they also do without gelatin, but eat products from live animals such as milk and honey.

Lacto-vegetarians avoid meat, fish and eggs.

Ovo vegetarians do without meat and fish as well as milk and milk products.

Pescetarians do not eat meat, but fish.

Fruitarians want plants to be harmed as little as possible. They mainly eat fruit and nuts.

Flexitarians are occasional vegetarians who value healthy food but do not continuously avoid meat or fish. (AP)

Tips to be successful at vegan diet

The reasons for a vegan diet are manifold: The motives range of health benefits on food intolerances to ethical and ideological considerations and the desire to protect the environment.

But those who eat free from animal foods such as eggs, dairy products and honey should note the following.

Vegan diet: easier than you think When switching to a vegan diet, the financial and time expenditure initially seems great. But vegan nutrition is neither more expensive nor takes more time than eating animal products.

Delicious recipes, forward-looking (shopping) planning, a pantry filled with basics - such as various types of grain, potatoes, pasta, rice and legumes - and a little bit of fun with the meal prep ensure little financial and time expenditure.

The vegan food pyramid

The vegan food pyramid consists of seven levels.

The basis is sufficient movement. Vegans should drink at least 1.5 liters of water a day. 250 g of fruit and 400 g of vegetables should be eaten daily. In addition, three portions of cereals and potatoes daily.

A serving of legumes and other protein sources should be on the table each day. Milk alternatives, nuts, seeds, oils and fats as well as seaweed provide many nutrients. At the top are alcohol, snacks and sweets: You can enjoy in moderation.

Vegan weekly menu

A vegan weekly menu is suitable for implementing a balanced, varied and healthy vegan diet - which also requires little time and money.

With the help of the vegan food pyramid and with the risk of a lack of nutrients in mind, the weekly schedule can be drawn up: once the basic structure is in place, dishes or individual components can be easily exchanged or replaced. An example of a vegan eating plan can be found at Peta 4. Sustainable vegan diet

Vegan diet uses less energy, resources and water than a diet with animal products. It leads to less animal suffering and leaves a smaller ecological footprint.

Nevertheless, the vegan diet is not automatically sustainable. Organic and fair products as well as a seasonal and regional orientation are crucial for a sustainable vegan diet.

Chapter 2: The Solution to Save Time and Money.

Meal prepping is about dedicating sufficient time to batch cook certain ingredients or prepare full meals for the week that lies ahead to make it easier to feed yourself as well as your family. It can be something as simple as preparing a sauce and chopping up a bunch of vegetables or as involved as cooking a full-fledged meal and then portioning it. If you want to get a head start on the week and reduce the time spent in the kitchen cooking, then meal prepping is quintessential.

There is no one size fits all kind of process involved in meal prepping. It differs from one person to another and from one household to another. Meal prepping does not necessarily mean preparing or prepping, cooking, and portioning every single meal you plan to consume in the following week. What might work for one person doesn't necessarily work for someone else. Also, the way you prepare meals will differ from one week to another, depending on the meals you wish to cook.

The terms meal prepping, and meal planning are often used synonymously, but they are not the same. These two techniques certainly make it easier to cook meals, but there are some differences. Meal prep is about setting a specific block of time aside to prep all the ingredients or cook meals for the week that lies ahead. On the other hand, meal planning essentially means planning the meals you wish to have. It is about answering the basic question of, "What's for dinner today?" These two tactics work hand-in-hand, and one cannot exist without the other.

Steps Involved in Meal Prep

Now that you know what meal prepping is, it is time to get started. There are three important steps involved in meal prep, and they are as follows.

Identifying your needs

Before you start prepping, you need to understand your needs and requirements. Meal prepping makes it easier to cook meals. So, what are the different things you will need to do to ensure you feel more in control of the food you eat? Think about all the pain points associated with mealtime. Do you need to cook a healthy lunch you can carry to work? Do you wish to stock up on vegan snacks? Do you want to stop spending a lot of money on breakfast?

Maybe you can start focusing by prepping ingredients required to whip up a quick breakfast in the morning. Perhaps you can start by prepping for lunch before anything else. Or maybe you want to quickly get the dinner ready and on the table within 20 minutes of reaching home. Once you identify the challenges involved, it is time to begin. Regardless of what you do, don't ever try to start prepping everything at once. Identify the biggest challenge, tackle it first, and then move onto something else. Once you get the hang of meal prepping, it becomes easier to cater to all your needs and requirements. So, start slowly and don't rush into it.

Selecting the right foods

Selecting the foods, you want to prep ahead to meet your needs is the second step. It certainly sounds quite easy, doesn't it? You might want to eat healthier breakfast, a light lunch, or perhaps a quick dinner. However, where do you start? Well, this is exactly where this book comes in. It presents plenty of meal prep ideas as well as recipes you can start using.

In general, there are two options available. Whenever you think about meal prepping, you can either opt for a recipe you can make ahead and store such as a batch of chili or your favorite curry. These can be repurposed for different meals. The second option is to mix and match components such as batch cooking roasted vegetables, whole grains, or even proteins like tofu.

Creating a plan

Once you are aware of all that you wish to cook ahead, this is what you will need to do next. Start making a list of all the tasks you want to accomplish within the meal prepping time you have set aside. Make a list of items you will need to cook and think of ways in which you can multitask. Perhaps you can cook something on the stovetop while another item is baking in the oven.

When the plan is ready, it is time to create a shopping list. It becomes easier to shop when you know all the ingredients you have to purchase.

Once you have completed both these steps, it is time to start prepping. Before you start prepping, ensure that you have set sufficient time aside for meal prep. Allocate anywhere between 2 to 4 hours during the weekend to prep meals for the upcoming week. Start with a clean kitchen; gather all the dishes you will need along with the equipment and the groceries, and start cooking. Maybe you can also turn on your favorite music to lift your spirits while prepping!

When all the prep is done, you must portion and store it! Store them in the right containers, label them if you want, and keep it in the fridge or the freezer. By following these steps, meal prepping will become incredibly simple. It will no longer seem overwhelming even if you never tried it before. All the effort that you put in will certainly be worth it.

Preparing and Storing Food

The idea of meal prepping and storing your prepped food can seem daunting and overwhelming. It might feel like you need lots of free time and lots of fancy kitchen equipment to get it done but that is far from the truth. Any and every one can meal prep so that they can reap the benefits, which include:

Ensuring that a minimal amount of time is spent in the kitchen.

Creating better productivity and efficiency because you do not have to spend time every day thinking about what you need to prepare to cook.

Sticking to a healthy lifestyle and diet since you no longer reach for unhealthy foods stemming from chronic exhaustion or a lack of willpower.

Keeping the cost of groceries down.

Reducing food wastage.

There are a few guidelines to help you get started on your vegan meal prepping and storage: Plan out your recipes. You can do this weekly or monthly. This allows you to also prepare a concise shopping list so that you buy exactly what you need and do not waste money on food that will not be eaten.

If you are a newbie vegan, start with the foods that you know and like. It is a great experiment however, you should start slowly, with foods and combos that you know while pairing them with individual new ingredients you would like to try out.

Make your own condiments. Many store-bought condiments are not vegan or ketogenic friendly. Therefore, the best option is to make your own condiments and sauces with ingredients that you know. These can usually be kept in the refrigerator for up to a week. You can find tasty sauce and condiment recipes in Chapter 5.

Make use of frozen produce. This can include frozen fruits and vegetables, which are usually cheap, fresh, and packed with a lot of nutrition. They also keep labor down to a minimum since no trimming or chopping is required and last longer since they are stored in the freezer.

Freezer versus refrigerator storage. Typically, food stored in the refrigerator needs to be eaten within three days, whereas food stored in the freezer lasts for up to six to eight months. If you store food in the freezer, be sure to take it out a day before so that you can eat it when you need to. Also, mark your food containers with dates to keep track of their expiry date.

Be careful with high protein foods to avoid food poisoning. Plant-based foods generally have lowered the risk of food poisoning compared to animal-based foods. However, bacteria thrive in protein-rich foods. Therefore, be sure to take extra care when storing and reheating these.

Be sure to always thoroughly reheat foods to avoid food poisoning. Never eat something that has just warmed as it may be in the food danger temperature zone where bacteria can thrive. Food that has been reheated needs to be extremely hot in the middle.

Never place warm food in the refrigerator. Allow food to cool completely before placing it in the refrigerator or freezer because you risk raising the internal temperature of the fridge which puts this item and other foods at risk for spoiling.

Defrost foods in a timely manner. Foods that have been frozen should be defrosted in the refrigerator or at room temperature before being eaten, typically at least 24 hours before consumption.

Benefits of Vegan Meal Prep

Who wouldn't want to lead a healthier life and feel more energized and fit? Well, everyone would want this. However, life can get a little hectic. Setting healthy goals is quite easy, but following through and staying on track becomes a little tricky. While you are busy navigating the hectic schedule of your daily life, the thought of cooking all your meals on your own is certainly not appealing. Not to mention the difficulty in thwarting off the temptations of eating out or ordering a meal. If you are tired of eating unhealthy junk food and want to eat healthier while saving some money, then meal prepping is the answer you have been looking for. In this section, let us look at some of the benefits of meal prep.

Grocery Shopping

Once you are aware of all the different meals you will be eating in a week, it becomes easier to shop for groceries. You no longer have to wander around aimlessly looking for inspiration or ideas to decide what to eat. Use the food list discussed in this book to prepare a grocery-shopping list. You can start dividing the list into different categories like vegetables, fruits, nuts and seeds, frozen foods, fats, and dairy alternatives. It also helps ensure that you don't give in to the temptation of buying unnecessary, processed foods.

Light on the Pocket

It is not expensive to start eating healthy. In fact, you might end up saving quite a lot of money. Once you start cooking all your meals at home. The only expenses you will incur are the ones towards shopping for groceries. Once you have everything you need to cook with, cooking becomes a breeze. Also, by planning all the meals, you will know what to buy and avoid making any unnecessary trips to the grocery store. When you know there is food waiting for you, it becomes easier to stop ordering meals.

Portion Control

An important skill you will learn once you start meal prepping is portion control. With meal prep, you will be dividing the food you cook into individual portions. By storing them in different containers, the urge to reach out for more or overindulge will be reduced. If weight loss is one of your priorities, then you need to consume sufficient nutrients. Portion control will help with this. You can certainly treat yourself occasionally, but learning to become mindful of the portions you eat is quintessential.

Healthy plant power without cholesterol

Foods with animal ingredients are often unhealthy. This is partly due to the mostly unhealthy preparation, but also due to the composition of animal products. Substances that are problematic to health, such as cholesterol, saturated fatty acids or purines, are increasingly found in animal products, while they are present in much smaller quantities or not at all in plants. In addition, many health-promoting ingredients, such as fiber and phytochemicals, are only ingested through plants.

No risk foods

When we attended the food safety training, we learned that food is divided into groups by the Health Department and assessed according to risk. Eggs, meat and fish are considered to be risky foods, and when they are prepared, increased safety requirements must be met. They are more susceptible to contamination. With one exception (sprouts), vegetable foods are not on this list. Your vegan meal prep is therefore longer-lasting and can also do without cooling for much longer.

Healthy with vegan foods

Many people find entry into the vegan diet due to health problems. In the case of numerous clinical pictures and complaints, a plant-based diet is recommended by doctors. Cancer patients are often advised to leave out milk products. Heart sufferers are advised not to eat meat. People with acne or neurodermatitis are also often advised not to eat milk products. A wholesome plant-based diet can also have a positive effect on blood, cholesterol and blood pressure values. If done correctly, the vegan diet and vegan meal prep can relieve symptoms and be used as a preventive measure. Some report having reached their ideal weight and positive effects on their digestion after changing their diet.

Improved sleep

Sleep is essential. Good sleep is essential, especially in a busy everyday life. Your body and mind need to regenerate at night and recharge your batteries. Since you cannot need long sleep or not sleep through! At this point, meal prep vegan comes in handy, because: Many types of vegetables and nuts contain vitamin B6, tryptophan and magnesium, which have a positive effect on sleep.

Ability to regenerate

Regeneration means "relaxation". The ability to regenerate is understood to mean the potential of humans to recover after physical and psychological stress. For example, a vegan diet can help regulate body weight. The "strength-to-body weight" can be influenced favorably, which improves sporting performance. The high proportion of valuable micronutrients in a balanced vegan diet is another reason why performance and the ability to regenerate can be improved. Another point why you should make your meal prep vegan

Weight Loss

When you know what you will be eating and how much you have to eat, you will automatically become mindful of the foods you consume. Weekly meal prep makes it easier to regulate the calories you consume daily. Since most of your meals will be home-cooked, you have complete control over the quality of ingredients you use. So, it is not just the quantity, but also the quality of the food you consume that improves as well. You don't necessarily have to count calories, but by substituting unhealthy ingredients with healthier alternatives, you can improve your overall health as well.

Less Wastage

Were there instances when you probably had to throw away produce because it expired or went bad before you had a chance to eat it? Wasting food is never a good feeling. It's not just a waste of money, but it is not environmentally sustainable. When you start meal prepping, you can make the most of all the ingredients you purchase. If you plan your meals correctly, you will be able to repurpose leftovers as well.

Saves Time and Effort

It does take a little time to plan and prepare meals in advance, but it is certainly worth the while. If you can dedicate a couple of hours over the weekend or whenever you are free to do the basic meal prep, cooking during the weekdays certainly becomes easier. Think about all the time you might usually end up worrying about what you will need to eat for your next meal. Once all your meals are prepared and planned, all that you need to do is reheat them and enjoy delicious and nutritious food.

Reduces Stress

Stress hurts your overall health. It not only weakens your immune system but also affects your sleeping pattern and digestive processes. Imagine how stressful it is when you come home after a hectic day and have to start thinking about what you need to eat for dinner. All this stress will be a thing of the past with meal prep. You can relax knowing that there is food ready when you go home.

Investment in Health

One of the great things about meal prep is that you can choose what you will be eating, and do this ahead of time. All those who follow meal prepping tend to eat cleaner than those who don't. You don't have to waste time finding something vegan to eat and risk eating unhealthy options because your meal is not ready. Eating healthy and well-balanced meals will undoubtedly improve your overall health. Proper nutrition is key to leading a healthy life.

Plenty of Variety

By putting a little thought into the kind of meals you will be eating, it becomes easier to select from different categories of foods like proteins, vegetables, fruits, and so on. When you plan, you can easily include the different food groups your body requires to all your meals. Apart from this, meal prep also encourages you to get creative with the recipes you use.

Better Willpower

Once you get into the groove of healthy eating, cravings for unhealthy foods and processed sugars will reduce. As your body gets used to the diet and the concept of healthy eating, it becomes easier to stay away from foods you know you must avoid.

Keep in mind that there is no right or wrong way to go about meal prepping. You have plenty of freedom to decide what you want to do. The best way to meal prep is via trial and error. After a week or two, you will quickly realize what works best for you.

Chapter 3: Macronutrient Intake

The macronutrients that constitute our diet are:

The Carbohydrates: also called carbon carbohydrates, sugars or more commonly, are the primary source of energy. They also contain the fibers, which we will define a little later.

The Fat: fatty acids also called "fat" or fat are molecules that form the organic fat. They play an important role in the constitution of cell membranes, energy production, and body temperature and more generally in the metabolism of the human being.

The Proteins: they are essential molecules for the life of cells and the constitution of human tissues (muscles, hair, skin, etc.).

Macronutrients are molecules that provide energy to our body or that participate directly or indirectly in metabolism. They are called "macro" in order to differentiate them from micronutrients such as vitamins, minerals, enzymes, etc.

Carbohydrates

It is the main source of energy of the body.

As you have guessed, it's about sugars, and yes sugars, we'll always need them. Everything depends then which sugars to privilege, and there, it becomes more complicated.

In theory, these are the complex sugars to favor at the expense of simple sugars, but that does not help you much!

What are the foods based on complex sugars and those based on simple sugars?

Simple sugars have a high glycemic index (Glucose and sucrose ...) they are present in sweets, pastries, classic white sugar, in many prepared dishes, sauces (ketchup, bbq sauce, sweet and sour) Complex sugars, meanwhile, have a low glycemic index; they are present in cereals (whole grains, attention!) and legumes.

Sugar in fruits is also an excellent source of energy, but we must not forget that fructose must first be treated in the liver before 'be used by the body, and it cannot be part of the complex sugars, it is a so-called fast sugar, but does not have a too high glycemic index, (IG: 20 against 100 for glucose), which differentiates it especially glucose classic is that the carbohydrate intake is supplemented with a contribution of fiber, minerals and vitamins.

THE PROTIDES

In common parlance we often tend to call them "proteins", but this is an abuse of language, and yes, in fact the protides is a sort of "family" grouping proteins, amino acids, and peptides.

When we talk about proteins "protiderotides" we immediately think of our muscles, and yes you know well they are made up, but we must not forget that they are also made of 70% water, moreover the water content of our body represents on average about 65% of our mass, small parenthesis Back to our proteins, except the muscles (myosin, actin, myoglobin) , they are also present in our hair, nail our skin (keratin), but also in our red blood cells (globin).

They provide a multitude of functions within the cells:

Cell renewal

Role of protection (hair, nails, skin)

Physiological functioning (information transmission, digestion, immune defense)

Secondary energy role (after carbohydrates)

and it is also our only source of nitrogen (essential for life), and yes, it is a present element to link amino acids to each other.

Proteins are of animal or vegetable origin (legumes, cereals)

Contrary to many received ideas, vegetable proteins are not of less good quality than animal proteins, on the contrary.

Indeed, animal proteins also contain so-called saturated fats (we'll talk about it later), favoring weight gain, cardiovascular risks and clot formation, on the contrary vegetable proteins are rich in fibers without any saturated fat.

How to calculate your own macros

It's about getting the right amount of each one right, so as not to fall short or exceed your body's needs. By achieving that balance, your body will function at its highest level and you will recover properly. It also activates other systems such as immune, digestive and sleep. "It's like a group of workers in which everyone does their job so that the whole body works at its maximum performance.

It is clear that this "work" depends on your level of activity and your objectives. "If you are an athlete, macros are very important. Also, if you eat adjusting to your macros, you don't have to eliminate any important food groups or deprive yourself of anything.

But if you want to lose fat, gain muscle, it is very important to consider the source and quality of the food you eat. "I have seen people who count macros stuffing themselves with donuts because 'it fits their macros', but they perform less and feel worse than if they had opted for sweet potatoes or other types of carbohydrates," he adds.

Tips for a healthy life through meal plan

Write your goals in our quadrant and with the tests in a visible place, start with a simple exercise routine, for example going for a walk

Eliminate sources of liquid calories, coffee, soda, alcohol, replace them with water, green tea and natural juices

Template to write what you eat (without forgetting anything)

Make your exercise day increasing the time and intensity of them

Change from 3 large meals to 6 small ones, each day adding fruit, vegetables and protein at all meals

Make a shopping list with healthy foods and go shopping with a full stomach, with a satiated appetite

Weigh yourself and write on a table as you move forward in your challenge

Choose an activity to do 3 times a week, it can be a sport, a dance class or just keep walking longer or with more intensity

Always plan the next week's menu

Add more fruit and vegetables to your diet than you have ever eaten before or long ago you eliminated from the diet

Make sure you are drinking enough water, about 8 glasses (2 liters of water per day approx)

Pay attention to the amount of fiber you consume per day, at least 35gr is recommended, if you do not reach this figure, consume some almonds (these will also help you control your appetite)

Chapter 4: Right Containers

Use proper storage containers. These should be BPA-free, microwavable, and dishwasher safe. Ziploc style bags are also great for storing food in the refrigerator and freezer and can be reused multiple times.

If you want to cook in batches or cook multiple portions of the same item, then you need to have the proper containers to store them. Keep in mind your favorite dishes while doing meal prep. Always opt for reusable containers instead of disposable ones. It certainly helps save time and money, not to mention that they are environment-friendly as well.

This is important for fresh food and economy. Cold storage equipment makes shopping easier and keeps food fresh. To take advantage of bargains in grocery and greengrocery, cold storage conditions are essential.

A cool, dry store cupboard with narrow 5-inch shelves taking single rows of tins, jars or packets. All groceries, even canned and processed foods keep best in a cool store, rather than a warm kitchen cupboard where they may lose their vitamin value.

A refrigerator as large as possible and with plenty of large containers with tight lids to keep fruit and vegetables fresh.

A deep freezer preferably 10-20 cubic feet. Choose a cupboard model or chest with a top opening and use a thermometer to check the temperature, which must be at 0°F. or − I 8°C. Store freshly baked bread, broths, doughs, prepared fruit and vegetables, ready-cooked dishes, pastry and soups, all tightly wrapped in special, heavy gauge polythene and closed to keep airtight.

6. Apparatuses and Gadgets

I'm very little of an apparatus and device individual. For me, the most significant apparatus is a nourishment processor as well as a fast blender. Contingent upon your financial limit, space, cooking needs and proclivity for machines, you may likewise need a submersion blender, a stand blender, a moderate cooker, a weight cooker, a rice cooker, and a waffle stove. Mainstream devices incorporate an electric can opener, a spiralizer for making veggie noodles, a pasta producer, hand blender, bread machines, juicers and frozen yogurt creators. It's a brilliant plan to just purchase what you truly require and have space for so you don't have a lot of devices occupying the room and gathering dust. I want to get things done by hand however that is my own inclination.

At the point when your kitchen is really, composed, productive, and well-supplied, it makes cooking to a greater extent a delight and to a lesser degree an errand. Rather than a room where work occurs, it turns into a sanctuary of imagination, motivation, and obviously, heavenliness. You may find that you can hardly wait to get into the kitchen and start making sound and delectable plant-based dishes.

Chapter 5: What Is Nutritious Vegan Food?

Foods to Avoid on the Vegan Diet

On a vegan diet, you should avoid consuming any animal foods or foods that contain ingredients that were derived from animals. The list of foods to avoid on a vegan diet include: • Poultry and meat. This includes organic meat, wild meat, chicken, turkey, duck, quail, beef, lamb, pork, veal, etc.

• Eggs. This can be from any animals including chickens, fish, ostriches, etc.

• Seafood and fish. This includes all types of fish and seafood including shrimp, squid, crab, lobster, mussels, anchovies, scallops, etc.

• Dairy products. This includes cheese, butter, cream, yogurt, milk, etc.

• Bee products. This includes honey, royal jelly, bee pollen, etc.

• Animal-based products. This list includes fish derived omega-3 fatty acids, animal derived vitamin D3, whey, lactose, egg white albumen, gelatin, shellac L-cysteine, casein, etc.

This list is pretty extensive but there are still some surprising foods that you may not realize are not vegan friendly. This list includes:

• Milk chocolate. Cocoa itself is vegan but milk, milk products, whey, and casein are often added to chocolate.

• Wine and beer. A gelatin-based substance which is derived from fish is often used as a clarifying agent in the manufacture of wine and beer.

• Sugar. Table sugar, which is made from sugar beets or sugarcane, is both completely fine to use. However, some sugars are processed with bone char, which is used in the refining process to help whiten sugar. Bone char is not vegan-friendly.

• Sugary snacks. Some of your favorite candies like gummies and marshmallows contain gelatin, which is derived from animals, and hence not vegan-friendly.

• Red processed foods. Some foods such as yogurt, fruit juices, soda, and candy contain an ingredient called carmine (otherwise known as red dye), which is derived from an insect.

• Non-dairy creamers. Some of these contain a milk-based derivative called sodium caseinate.

• Worcestershire sauce. Traditional recipes for this include anchovies. Note that there are vegan-friendly options available.

• Bread. Many common bread options include egg, butter, milk and other animal byproducts in the ingredient list. Luckily, there are bread recipes available which do not contain such ingredients.

• Omega-3 fortified products. Ensure that the packaging for your omega-3 fortified purchases do not contain fish-based ingredients like sardines, anchovies, and tilapia.

Foods to Eat on the Vegan Diet

This list includes plant and plant-based products such as:

• Fruits and vegetables

• Whole grains, cereals, and pseudo-cereals such as spelt, quinoa, and teff—all of which are high-protein options that are also great sources of complex carbs, B vitamins, and several minerals such as zinc, iron, potassium, to name a few, and fiber.

• Fermented and sprouted plant foods. This includes pickles, kimchi, Ezekiel bread, miso, natto, and tempeh.

• Nutritional yeast. This is a great protein supplement you can include in dishes as a substitute for cheese given its cheesy flavor.

• Seeds such as chia seeds, flax seeds, and hemp seeds which are good sources of protein and omega-3 fatty acids.

• Nuts and nut butters are great sources of fiber, magnesium, zinc, selenium, vitamin E, and iron. The unroasted and unblanched varieties are best.

• Legumes such as lentils, beans, and peas are great protein sources and increase nutrient absorption.

• Plant-based protein replacements. This includes tofu, tempeh, and seitan. They make great replacements for meat, fish, poultry, and eggs in recipes.

• Calcium-fortified plant milks and yogurts. These are a great replacement for milk and yogurt and help provide the recommended daily supplement of calcium. Try to get versions that have been fortified with vitamin B12 and D when possible.

Some vegans we find it difficult to ensure that they get adequate supplies of all nutrients required daily. Therefore, supplements can be taken to fortify the vegan diet. Supplements include EPA and DHA, which are omega-3 fatty acids which can be sourced from algae oil, Iron, vitamin D, vitamin B12, calcium, zinc and iodine, which can also be supplemented by adding 1/2 teaspoon of iodized salt to your diet.

Eating Out on a Vegan Diet

Eating out on any diet can be challenging and the same can be said for eating out as a vegan. The way to make this as stress-free as possible for you is to plan ahead. To make this process easier for you, here are a few tips that you can employ while eating out:

• Try to find the restaurant menu online beforehand so that you can determine if there are any vegan options available.

• You may try calling ahead to arrange a special vegan dish with the chef.

• At the restaurants, you can simply ask the staff about any vegan options available before you get seated so that you can know if this restaurant is the right choice for you.

• Try ethnic restaurants such as Mexican, Thai, Indian, Middle-Eastern, and Ethiopian cuisine because they tend to have several natural vegan-friendly options.

• At a restaurant, try to identify the vegetarian options on the menu and ask if any dairy or egg products can be removed to make the dish vegan-friendly.

• If there are no vegan meal options, order several vegan appetizers or side dishes to make up a meal.

• Also check out the new vegetarian and vegan restaurants within your neighborhood. With the widespread awareness of leading a plant-based lifestyle gaining traction each day, there are always newer pure vegan and vegetarian restaurants also popping up everywhere you go!

Chapter 6: Breakfast

Green Kickstart Smoothie

Preparation time: 5 minutes

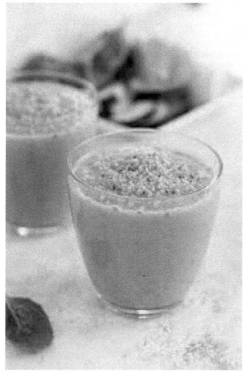

Servings: 1

Ingredients

½ Avocado or 1 banana

½ Cup chopped cucumber, peeled if desired

1 handful fresh spinach or chopped lettuce

1 pear or apple, peeled and cored, or 1 cup unsweetened applesauce

2 tablespoons freshly squeezed lime juice

1 cup water or nondairy milk, plus more as needed

Additions

½-Inch piece peeled fresh ginger

1 tablespoon ground flaxseed or chia seeds

½ Cup soy yogurt or 3 ounces silken tofu

Coconut water to replace some of the liquid

2 tablespoons chopped fresh mint or ½ cup chopped mango

Directions:

In a blender, combine the avocado, cucumber, spinach, pear, lime juice, and water.

Add any Additions Ingredients as desired. Purée until smooth and creamy, about 50 seconds. Add a bit more water if you like a thinner smoothie.

Nutrition: calories: 263; protein: 4g; total fat: 14g; saturated fat: 2g; carbohydrates: 36g; fiber: 10g

Warm Quinoa Breakfast Bowl

Preparation time: 5 minutes

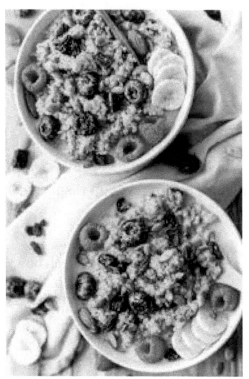

Cooking time: 0 minutes

Servings: 4

Ingredients

3 cups freshly cooked quinoa

1⅓ cups unsweetened soy or almond milk

2 bananas, sliced

1 cup raspberries

1 cup blueberries

½ Cup chopped raw walnuts

¼ Cup maple syrup

Directions:

Divide the Ingredients among 4 bowls, starting with a base of ¾ cup quinoa, ⅓ cup milk, ½ banana, ¼ cup raspberries, ¼ cup blueberries, and 2 tablespoons walnuts.

Drizzle 1 tablespoon of maple syrup over the top of each bowl.

Banana Bread Rice Pudding

Preparation time: 5 minutes

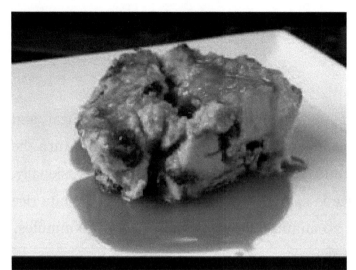

Cooking time: 50 minutes

Servings: 4

Ingredients

1cup brown rice

1½ cups water

1½ cups nondairy milk

3 tablespoons sugar (omit if using a sweetened nondairy milk)

2 teaspoons pumpkin pie spice or ground cinnamon

2 bananas

3 tablespoons chopped walnuts or sunflower seeds (optional)

Directions

In a medium pot, combine the rice, water, milk, sugar, and pumpkin pie spice. Bring to a boil over high heat, turn the heat to low, and cover the pot. Simmer, stirring occasionally, until the rice is soft and the liquid is absorbed. White rice takes about 20 minutes; brown rice takes about 50 minutes.

Smash the bananas and stir them into the cooked rice. Serve topped with walnuts (if using). Leftovers will keep refrigerated in an airtight container for up to 5 days.

Nutrition: calories: 479; protein: 9g; total fat: 13g; saturated fat: 1g; carbohydrates: 86g; fiber: 7g

Apple and cinnamon oatmeal

Preparation time: 10 minutes

Cooking time:10 minutes

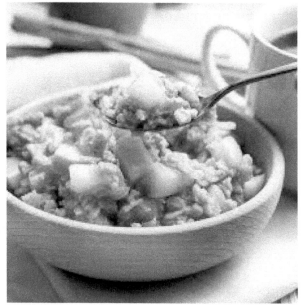

Servings: 2

Ingredients

1¼ cups apple cider

1 apple, peeled, cored, and chopped

⅔ Cup rolled oats

1 teaspoon ground cinnamon

1 tablespoon pure maple syrup or agave (optional)

Directions

In a medium saucepan, bring the apple cider to a boil over medium-high heat. Stir in the apple, oats, and cinnamon.

Bring the cereal to a boil and turn down heat to low. Simmer until the oatmeal thickens, 3 to 4 minutes. Spoon into two bowls and sweeten with maple syrup, if using. Serve hot.

Spiced orange breakfast couscous

Preparation time: 10 minutes

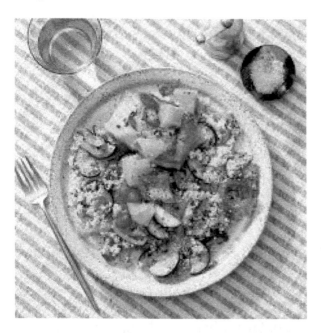

Cooking time: 10 minutes

Servings: 4

Ingredients

3 cups orange juice

1½ cups couscous

1 teaspoon ground cinnamon

¼ Teaspoon ground cloves

½ Cup dried fruit, such as raisins or apricots

½ Cup chopped almonds or other nuts or seeds

Directions

In a small saucepan, bring the orange juice to a boil. Add the couscous, cinnamon, and cloves and remove from heat. Cover the pan with a lid and allow to sit until the -couscous softens, about 5 minutes.

Fluff the couscous with a fork and stir in the dried fruit and nuts. Serve -immediately.

Nutrition: calories 120, fat 1, fiber 2, carbs 3, protein 5

Breakfast parfaits

Preparation time: 15 minutes

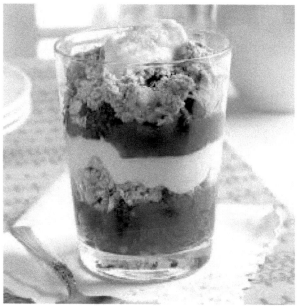

Cooking time: 0 minutes

Servings: 2

Ingredients

One 14-ounce can coconut milk, refrigerated overnight

1 cup granola

½ Cup walnuts

1 cup sliced strawberries or other seasonal berries

Directions

Pour off the canned coconut-milk liquid and retain the solids.

In two parfait glasses, layer the coconut-milk solids, granola, walnuts, and -strawberries. Serve immediately.

Nutrition: calories 100, fat 1, fiber 2, carbs 3, protein 5

Sweet potato and kale hash

Preparation time: 10 minutes

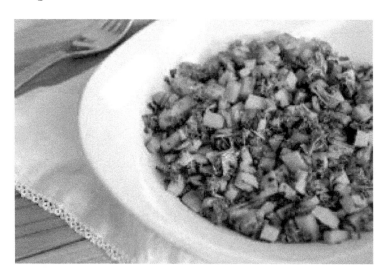

Cooking time: 15 minutes

Servings: 2

Ingredients

1 sweet potato

2 tablespoons olive oil

½ Onion, chopped

1 carrot, peeled and chopped

2 garlic cloves, minced

½ Teaspoon dried thyme

1 cup chopped kale

Sea salt

Freshly ground black pepper

Directions

Prick the sweet potato with a fork and microwave on high until soft, about 5 minutes. Remove from the microwave and cut into ¼-inch cubes.

In a large nonstick sauté pan, heat the olive oil over medium-high heat. Add the onion and carrot and cook until softened, about 5 minutes. Add the garlic and thyme and cook until the garlic is fragrant, about 30 seconds.

Add the sweet potatoes and cook until the potatoes begin to brown, about 7 -minutes. Add the kale and cook just until it wilts, 1 to 2 minutes. Season with salt and pepper. Serve immediately.

Nutrition: calories 90, fat 1, fiber 2, carbs 3, protein 5

Delicious Oat Meal

Preparation time: 10 minutes

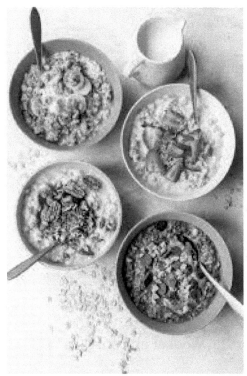

Cooking time: 6 hours

Servings: 4

Ingredients:

3 cups water

3 cups almond milk

1 and ½ cups steel oats

4 dates, pitted and chopped

1 teaspoon cinnamon, ground

2 tablespoons coconut sugar

½ Teaspoon ginger powder

A pinch of nutmeg, ground

A pinch of cloves, ground

1 teaspoon vanilla extract

Directions:

Put water and milk in your slow cooker and stir.

Add oats, dates, cinnamon, sugar, ginger, nutmeg, cloves and vanilla extract, stir, cover and cook on low for 6 hours.

Divide into bowls and serve for breakfast.

Enjoy!

Nutrition: calories 120, fat 1, fiber 2, carbs 3, protein 5

Breakfast Cherry Delight

Preparation time: 10 minutes

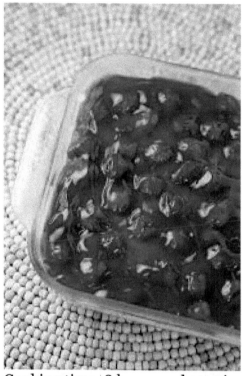

Cooking time: 8 hours and 10 minutes

Servings: 4

Ingredients:

2 cups almond milk

2 cups water

1 cup steel cut oats

2 tablespoons cocoa powder

1/3 cup cherries, pitted

¼ Cup maple syrup

½ Teaspoon almond extract

For the sauce:

2 tablespoons water

1 and ½ cups cherries, pitted and chopped

¼ Teaspoon almond extract

Directions:

Put the almond milk in your slow cooker.

Add 2 cups water, oats, cocoa powder, 1/3 cup cherries, maples syrup and ½ teaspoon almond extract.

Stir, cover and cook on low for 8 hours.

In a small pan, mix 2 tablespoons water with 1 and ½ cups cherries and ¼ teaspoon almond extract, stir well, bring to a simmer over medium heat and cook for 10 minutes until it thickens.

Divide oatmeal into breakfast bowls, top with the cherries sauce and serve.

Enjoy!

Nutrition: calories 150, fat 1, fiber 2, carbs 6, protein 5

Crazy Maple and Pear Breakfast

Preparation time: 10 minutes

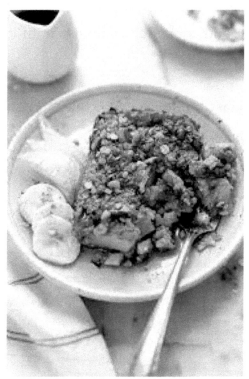

Cooking time: 9 hours

Servings: 2

Ingredients:

1 pear, cored and chopped

½ Teaspoon maple extract

2 cups coconut milk

½ Cup steel cut oats

½ Teaspoon vanilla extract

1 tablespoon stevia

¼ Cup walnuts, chopped for serving

Cooking spray

Directions:

Spray your slow cooker with some cooking spray and add coconut milk.

Also, add maple extract, oats, pear, stevia and vanilla extract, stir, cover and cook on low for 9 hours.

Stir your oatmeal again, divide it into breakfast bowls and serve with chopped walnuts on top.

Enjoy!

Nutrition: calories 150, fat 3, fiber 2, carbs 6, protein 6

Hearty French Toast Bowls

Preparation time: 10 minutes

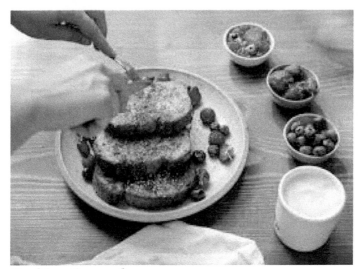

Cooking time: 5 hours

Servings: 4

Ingredients:

1 and ½ cups almond milk

1 cup coconut cream

1 tablespoon vanilla extract

½ Tablespoon cinnamon powder

2 tablespoons maple syrup

¼ Cup spend

2 apples, cored and cubed

½ Cup cranberries, dried

1-pound vegan bread, cubed

Cooking spray

Directions:

Spray your slow cooker with some cooking spray and add the bread.

Also, add cranberries and apples and stir gently.

Add milk, coconut cream, maple syrup, vanilla extract, cinnamon powder and splenda.

Stir, cover and cook on low for 5 hours.

Divide into bowls and serve right away.

Enjoy!

Nutrition: calories 140, fat 2, fiber 3, carbs 6, protein 2

Tofu Burrito

Preparation time: 10 minutes

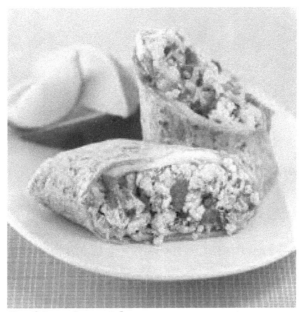

Cooking time: 8 hours

Servings: 4

Ingredients:

15 ounces canned black beans, drained

2 tablespoons onions, chopped

7 ounces tofu, drained and crumbled

2 tablespoons green bell pepper, chopped

½ Teaspoon turmeric

¾ Cup water

¼ Teaspoon smoked paprika

¼ Teaspoon cumin, ground

¼ Teaspoon chili powder

A pinch of salt and black pepper

4 gluten free whole wheat tortillas

Avocado, chopped for serving

Salsa for serving

Directions:

Put black beans in your slow cooker.

Add onions, tofu, bell pepper, turmeric, water, paprika, cumin, chili powder, a pinch of salt and pepper, stir, cover and cook on low for 8 hours.

Divide this on each tortilla, add avocado and salsa, wrap, arrange on plates and serve.

Enjoy!

Nutrition: calories 130, fat 4, fiber 2, carbs 5, protein 4

Tasty Mexican Breakfast

Preparation time: 10 minutes

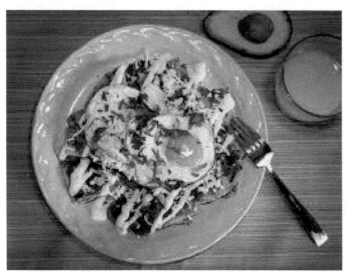

Cooking time: 2 hours

Servings: 4

Ingredients:

1 cup brown rice

1 cup onion, chopped

2 cups veggie stock

1 red bell pepper, chopped

1 green bell pepper, chopped

4 ounces canned green chilies, chopped

15 ounces canned black beans, drained

A pinch of salt

Black pepper to the taste

For the salsa:

3 tablespoons lime juice

1 avocado, pitted, peeled and cubed

½ Cup cilantro, chopped

½ Cup green onions, chopped

½ Cup tomato, chopped

1 poblano pepper, chopped

2 tablespoons olive oil

½ Teaspoon cumin

Directions:

Put the stock in your slow cooker.

Add rice, onions and beans, stir, cover and cook on high for 1 hour and 30 minutes.

Add chilies, red and green bell peppers, a pinch of salt and black pepper, stir, cover again and cook on high for 30 minutes more.

Meanwhile, in a bowl, mix avocado with green onions, tomato, poblano pepper, cilantro, oil, cumin, a pinch of salt, black pepper and lime juice and stir really well.

Divide rice mix into bowls; top each with the salsa you've just made and serve.

Enjoy!

Nutrition: calories 140, fat 2, fiber 2, carbs 5, protein 5

Chapter 7: Lunch Recipes

Herby Giant Couscous with Asparagus and Lemon

Preparation time: 5 minutes

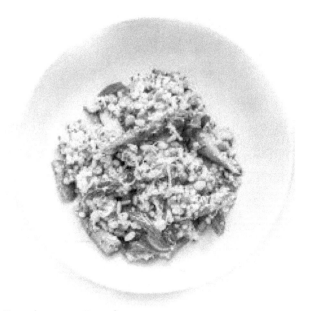

Servings: 2 Servings

Ingredients

150 g giant couscous

100 g asparagus tips

100 g frozen peas

3 tbsp. walnut oil

Juice and zest of 1 lemon

Handful fresh parsley

Handful of fresh mint

Handful baby spinach

2 tbsp. pine nuts

Direction

Bring a large pot of salted water to a boil. Add giant couscous. After 5 minutes, add asparagus and peas and boil for another 4 minutes.

While the couscous is cooking, cook in a mini blender (or directly in a bowl, sharp knife and elbow grease!), Walnut oil, lemon juice, parsley, and mint.

Drain the couscous and immediately stir the dressing of the baby herb and spinach.

Divide between two plates and crush with pine nuts and lemon lotion.

Nutrition: calories: 263; protein: 4g; total fat: 14g; saturated fat: 2g; carbohydrates: 36g; fiber: 10g

Veggieful' Chili

Servings: 8

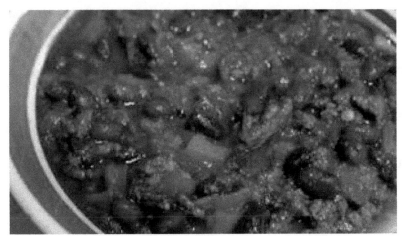

Preparation Time: 15 minutes

Ingredients:

1½ cups raw black beans

1½ cups raw kidney beans

2 tbsp. olive oil

2 red onions (medium, diced)

1 clove garlic (minced)

2 tsp. cumin

¼ tsp. cayenne pepper

2 tsp. oregano

1 zucchini (medium, diced)

1 yellow squash (small, diced)

1 red bell pepper (small, diced)

2 cups water

1 jalapeño (medium, diced)

1 cup tomato paste

1 (200g) can sweet corn (drained)

1 tbsp. chili powder

Salt and pepper to taste

Directions:

Prepare the black and kidney beans according to the Directions.

Take a large pan, put it on medium high heat and add the olive oil.

Sautee the diced red onions for about 5 minutes.

Blend in the garlic, cumin, cayenne pepper, oregano while stirring.

Add the diced zucchini, squash, bell pepper and stir again.

Allow the mixture to fry for a few minutes while constantly stirring.

Lower the heat to medium and add 2 cups of water, jalapeño, tomato paste, corn and cooked beans.

Stir well while adding the chili powder, salt and optionally more pepper to taste.

Reduce the heat to low, cover the pan and let the chili simmer for about 20 minutes.

Add more spices like cumin, oregano, chili powder or cayenne pepper to taste.

Serve and enjoy warm or allow the chili to cool down to store it in containers!

Nutrition:

Calories: 256 kcal.

Carbs: 43.6g.

Fat: 4.5gr.

Protein: 13g.

Fiber: 16.8g.

Sugar: 8.5g.

Red Curry Lentils

Servings: 6

Preparation Time: 20 minutes

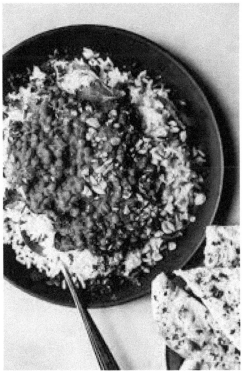

Ingredients:

1 cup dry red lentils

2 tbsp. coconut oil

1 tbsp. cumin seeds

1 tbsp. coriander seeds

8 tomatoes (ripe, cubed)

1 head of garlic (chopped or minced)

2 tbsp. ginger (chopped)

1 tbsp. turmeric

1 tsp. cayenne powder

3 cups vegetable broth

2 tsp. sea salt

1 (15oz.) can coconut milk

½ cup cherry tomatoes

½ cup cilantro (chopped)

Directions:

Soak and drain the red lentils according to the Directions but do not cook them yet.

Put the coconut oil in a large pot heating over medium high heat.

Add the cumin and coriander seeds and garlic. Sauté the Ingredients for about 2 minutes while continuously stirring.

Add the freshly cut tomato cubes, ginger, turmeric and a pinch of salt to the pot.

Allow the mixture to gently cook, stirring occasionally for 5 minutes.

Blend in the red lentils, more salt to taste and cayenne powder.

Continue to add 3 cups of vegetable broth to the pot and allow the mixture to come to a soft boil.

Reduce the heat to low, cover the pot and allow the dish to simmer for about 30 minutes while stirring occasionally.

Once the lentils are soft, add the coconut milk and cherry tomatoes.

Bring the mixture back to a simmer before removing it from the heat and stir in the chopped cilantro.

Serve warm or allow the curry to cool down before storing.

Nutrition:

Calories: 162 kcal.

Carbs: 19.3g.

Fat: 6.8g.

Protein: 6g.

Fiber: 6.5g.

Sugar: 5.8g.

Black-Bean Veggie Burritos

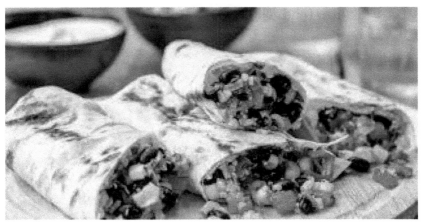

Servings: 8

Preparation Time: 30 minutes

Ingredients

For the filling:

2 cups dry black beans

1 tbsp. olive oil

1 red onion (diced)

1 zucchini (cubed)

1 red bell pepper (pitted, diced)

2 (150g) cans sweet corn (drained, rinsed)

¼ cup cilantro (chopped)

½ a lime (juiced)

Salt to taste

For homemade taco seasoning (optional)

1 tbsp. chili powder

2 tsp. ground cumin

½ tsp. paprika powder

¼ tsp. of each: garlic powder, onion powder, red pepper flakes, oregano, salt and cayenne

For the wraps:

8 tortilla wraps

½ cup no-salt vegan cream cheese

½ cup salsa

1 cup dry brown rice

Directions:

Cook the black beans according to the Directions.

Prepare the brown rice according to the recipe.

Mix all taco seasoning Ingredients in a bowl and set it aside.

Take a large pan, add the olive oil and put it on medium heat.

Add the diced red onion. Sauté for 3 minutes while stirring.

Add the zucchini and bell pepper and sauté for another 3 minutes.

Add in the black beans, corn and the homemade taco seasoning. Stir well and allow the mixture to simmer for about 10 minutes.

Turn off the heat and add the cilantro, lime juice and salt to taste.

Prepare the burrito by laying out a tortilla wrap and add the filling, salsa, rice and the optional vegan cheese.

Tightly wrap the burrito and place it back in the pan. Heat and press each side for about 2 minutes.

Serve warm or store each tortilla wrapped in aluminum foil in a Ziploc bag.

Nutrition:

Calories: 285 kcal.

Carbs: 40.9g.

Fat: 9.8g.

Protein: 8.6g.

Fiber: 6.7g.

Sugar: 4.3g.

Baked Red Bell Peppers

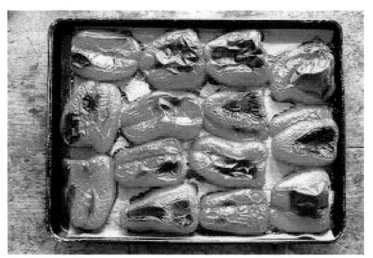

Servings: 8

Preparation Time: 30 minutes

Ingredients:

1 cup dry chickpeas

1½ cup dry quinoa

4 red bell peppers (seeded, halved lengthwise)

1½ tbsp. olive oil

1 red onion (medium, diced)

1 clove garlic (medium, minced)

2 tbsp. chili powder

2 tsp. cumin

1 tsp. cayenne pepper

2 tsp. spicy paprika powder

2 cups baby spinach (chopped)

3 tomatoes (ripe, medium, chopped)

¼ cup fresh cilantro (chopped)

Salt and pepper to taste

Directions:

Preheat the oven to 375°F or 190°C.

Prepare the chickpeas according to the Directions.

Prepare the quinoa according to the recipe.

Put the olive oil into a skillet on medium heat.

Sautee the diced red onions until soft.

Add the garlic, chili powder, cumin, cayenne pepper, paprika powder, salt and pepper to the skillet and stir everything for about 2 minutes.

Stir in the remaining Ingredients except the cilantro and add more salt and pepper to taste.

Heat the stuffing for another 5 minutes until the Ingredients are browned.

Turn off the heat, add dd the cilantro and divide the stuffing into the halved red bell peppers.

Put the peppers on a lightly greased baking tray and cover them with aluminum foil.

Place the tray in the oven for about 20 to 25 minutes.

Take the tray out and allow the bell peppers to sit for about 5 minutes.

Serve right away or allow the stuffed red bell peppers to cool down for storage!

Nutrition:

Calories: 135 kcal.

Carbs: 20g.

Fat: 4g.

Protein: 4.5g.

Fiber: 16.4g.

Sugar: 5.5g.

Quick Quinoa Casserole

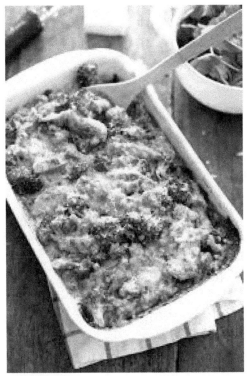

Servings: 9

Preparation Time: 15 minutes

Ingredients:

2 cups dry pinto beans

1 cup dry quinoa

1 (7 oz.) pack tempeh (sliced)

2 tbsp. olive oil

2 tsp. cumin

2 tsp. paprika powder

1 cup red onion (diced)

2 garlic cloves (minced)

6 sweet red peppers (small, sliced)

2 (4 oz.) cans green chilies (diced)

1 cup Roma tomatoes (diced)

2 cups vegetable broth

Salt and pepper to taste

½ cup no-salt cream cheese

1 avocado (diced, sliced or mashed)

¼ cup green onions (diced)

¼ cup cilantro (chopped, fresh)

Directions:

Cook the pinto beans according to the recipe.

Put a large skillet greased with the olive oil over medium heat.

Grill the tempeh slices with a tsp. paprika powder, cumin and salt and pepper to taste for about 5 minutes.

Take out the grilled tempeh slices and leave it aside.

Grease the same skillet with olive oil and sauté the onions.

Add the minced garlic while stirring.

Blend in the red peppers and stir the Ingredients for about 2 minutes.

Continue to add the green chilies, cooked pinto beans and quinoa, tomatoes and vegetable broth to the pan along with another tsp. of paprika powder, cumin, salt and pepper to taste.

Let the mixture cook for about 5 minutes.

Add the tempeh back to the skillet, stir, cover and reduce the heat to low.

Cook the mixture for about 15 minutes until the quinoa is soft and most of the broth has been absorbed.

Remove the skillet from the heat and add vegan cream cheese.

Put the lid on the skillet and let the dish sit for a minute until the cheese has melted.

Serve the quick quinoa casserole with fresh avocado slices, green onions and fresh cilantro.

Enjoy or store!

Nutrition:

Calories: 236 kcal.

Carbs: 24.9g.

Fat: 11g.

Protein: 9.2g.

Fiber: 7.4g.

Sugar: 4g.

Mexican Casserole

Servings: 4

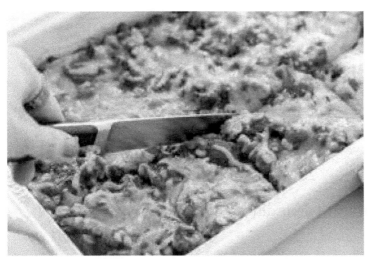

Preparation Time: 30 minutes

Ingredients:

1 cup dry black beans

1 cup dry white beans

1 tsp. olive oil

3 tbsp. Mexican spice

2 cups Mexican salsa

1½ cups cashew cheese spread

3 bell peppers (red and yellow, chopped)

1 red onion (chopped)

1 green onion (chopped)

1 jalapeno pepper (medium, seeded and chopped)

Salt and pepper to taste

Directions:

Cook the beans according to the Directions.

Preheat oven at 350°F or 175°C.

Grease a saucepan with the olive oil. Add Mexican spice, 1 cup of Mexican salsa and stir well.

Stir in the cashew cheese, chopped bell peppers, onions and add salt and pepper to taste.

Spread ½ cup salsa over the bottom of a casserole dish. Add the beans on top of the salsa and spread out the saucepan mix evenly over the beans.

Add the last ½ cup salsa sauce on top and sprinkle some chopped jalapenos on top.

Bake the casserole for 15-20 minutes.

Enjoy the dish after a short cooling period or let it cool down completely for storing.

Nutrition:

Calories: 442 kcal.

Carbs: 65.9g.

Fat: 11.5g.

Protein: 20.2g.

Fiber: 33.9g.

Sugar: 17.4g.

Mushroom Ragout

Servings: 10

Preparation Time: 45 minutes

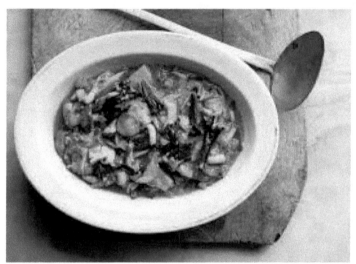

Ingredients:

2 tbsp. olive oil

1 sweet onion (large, finely chopped)

1 clove garlic (minced)

6 cups Portobello mushrooms (chopped)

½ cup dry red wine

1 cup vegetable broth

½ tbsp. nutritional yeast

¼ cup basil leaves (chopped)

¼ cup no-salt cream cheese substitute with cashew butter

¼ cup parsley (optional, chopped)

Salt and pepper to taste

Directions:

Take a large pot and put it on medium heat.

Sauté the onions and garlic in the olive oil while stirring.

Add some salt and pepper to taste and stir.

Mix in the mushrooms and turn up the heat a bit.

Cook and stir the mushrooms until most of the liquid in it has evaporated.

Add the red wine. Turn the heat up to medium-high and cook the ragout until most of the wine is evaporated.

Add the vegetable broth and stir thoroughly.

Blend in the nutritional yeast and cook the ragout for about 5 minutes.

Add the chopped basil and the no-salt cream cheese.

Lower the heat and keep stirring until the ragout simmers.

Keep stirring occasionally for about 5 more minutes and add more salt and pepper to taste.

Turn the heat off and set aside for about minutes to let the ragout cool down a bit.

Garnish with the optional parsley before serving and enjoy while warm or store.

Nutrition:

Calories: 77 kcal.

Carbs: 4.2g.

Fat: 4.1g.

Protein: 2.5g.

Fiber: 1.6g.

Sugar: 2.2g.

Pumpkin Pilaf

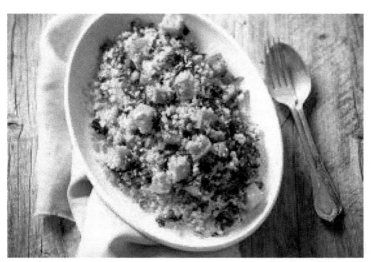

Servings: 2

Preparation Time: 20 minutes

Ingredients:

2 cup dry brown rice

2 tbsp. olive oil

1 sweet potato (medium, cubed)

2 cups fresh pumpkin (cubed)

2 cups kale (fresh or frozen)

2 celery ribs (medium, cut)

1 onion (medium, cut)

2 garlic cloves

1 tbsp. onion powder

1 bay leaf (chopped)

Salt and black pepper to taste

½ cup pumpkin seeds (optional)

Handful of fresh parsley (chopped, optional)

Directions:

Cook the rice according to the recipe.

Put a large skillet on medium heat and add the olive oil to the skillet.

Throw in the sweet potato and pumpkin cubes.

Add the kale, onion, celery, garlic and onion powder.

Cook the mixture for 15-20 minutes and turn the heat down to low.

Add the cooked rice, optional pumpkin seeds, a handful of fresh parsley and stir thoroughly.

Softly cook the mixture for another 5 minutes.

Enjoy or store the pilaf for another day!

Nutrition:

Calories: 557 kcal.

Carbs: 90.1g.

Fat: 16,8g.

Protein: 11.5g.

Fiber: 12.5g.

Sugar: 13.1g.

Chapter 8: Dinner Recipes

Baked Root Veg with Chili

Preparation time: 20 minutes

Servings: 2

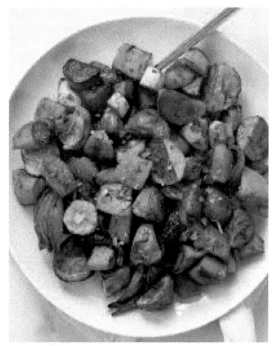

Ingredients:

Potatoes (three medium)

Sweet potato (three medium)

Yam (three small)

Vegetable broth (two cups)

Red kidney beans (one can)

White kidney beans (one can)

Diced tomatoes (two cans)

Black beans (one can)

Dried oregano (one teaspoon)

Paprika (one and a half teaspoons)

Cumin (two teaspoons)

Chili powder (two tablespoons)

Celery (two stalks)

Carrots (two medium)

Bell pepper (one large red)

Red onion (two medium)

Olive oil (two tablespoons)

Cilantro (one bunch)

Avocado (two medium)

Bay leaf (one leaf)

Sweet corn (one can)

Tomato (two medium)

Lime juice (two medium)

Romaine (one head)

Directions:

Scrub and fork the potatoes and yams. Drizzle them with oil and quickly run over with clean hands. Sprinkle with salt and put on a baking tray for forty-five minutes or until you can pierce easily with a knife.

Heat the oil in a frying pan on medium and add the diced onion with the chopped bell pepper, diced carrots, and celery along with a quarter teaspoon of salt. Cook until the carrot is tender then add the paprika, oregano, cumin, and chili powder, along with the finely diced garlic.

Put in the full contents of the tomato cans, the bay leaf, and the vegetable broth.

Rinse all the cans of beans and drain well before adding to the pot. Stir the pot well and leave to simmer for a further thirty minutes. After this time has passed, get a potato masher and mash the chili to squish some of the beans and thicken the mixture.

At this point, you can add the juice of one lime, and salt and pepper to taste.

In separate bowls, prepare the fresh ingredients: finely dice the avocado and lightly mash with salt, pepper and the juice of another lime. Drain and rinse the corn and toss with half of the cilantro, finely chopped. Shred the romaine lettuce and dice the tomatoes.

Check that the root vegetables are done, remove from oven and slice open to cool slightly. Place in a nice dish and put on the table with a bowl of chili and all the sides for people to build their own masterpiece. You may also want to get vegan sour cream for this meal from the store. Enjoy!

Nutrition: calories: 63; protein: 4g; total fat: 14g; saturated fat: 2g; carbohydrates: 36g; fiber: 10g

Autumn Stuffed Enchiladas

Preparation time: 20 minutes

Servings: 2

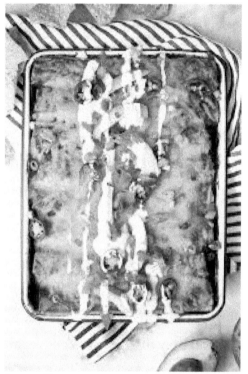

Ingredients:

Salt and pepper (to taste)

Lemon juice (one medium lemon)

Cashews (one cup raw)

Cilantro (one bunch)

Roasted pumpkin seeds (quarter cup)

Corn tortillas (twelve pack)

Butternut squash (two cups)

Salsa (one and a half cups homemade or store-bought)

Black beans (one can)

Olive oil (two tablespoons)

Cayenne pepper (quarter teaspoon)

Chili flakes (one teaspoon)

Cumin (one teaspoon)

Garlic (three cloves)

Jalapeno (one medium)

Red onion (one small)

Brussel sprouts (one cup)

Direction:

Soak the cashews in boiled water to cover and set aside.

Cut the squash in half and after scooping out the seeds, lightly rub olive oil with clean hands over the exposed flesh. Sprinkle with a little salt and pepper before putting on a baking sheet face down. Cook for about forty-five minutes at 400F until it is cooked through.

Heat one tablespoon of olive oil in a frypan on medium heat and put chopped onion in, stirring until soft. Finely dice the jalapeno and garlic and finely slice the Brussel sprouts. Add these three things to the frypan and cook until the Brussels begin to wilt through.

Strain and rinse the black beans then add those to the frypan and mix well.

When the squash is cooked through and cool enough to handle, scrape out the soft insides away from the skin and put in a big bowl along with the Brussels mixture. Mix well again with the addition of generous pinches of salt and pepper to taste)

Put the tortillas in the oven to soften up (don't let them get crispy) while you get a baking dish out and very lightly oil the base and sides before spooning some salsa into it and doing the same. Spoon the squash mixture into the middle of the soft tortillas. Carefully roll them up to make little open-ended wraps, then put in the baking dish with the open ends down to stop them from unrolling.

Do this for all twelve tortillas then pour the rest of the salsa on top and spread to evenly coat. Change the temperature of the oven to 350F and bake for thirty minutes.

While these cooks put the drained, soaked cashews into a blender with one and a half cups cold water, lemon juice, and a quarter teaspoon salt. Blend until smooth, adding tiny drizzles of water if it becomes too thick. This is your sour cream.

When enchiladas are done, leave to cool while you chop cilantro. Then drizzle the sour cream generously over the dish and top with cilantro and pumpkin seeds. Enjoy!

Nutrition: calories: 123; protein: 4g; total fat: 11g; saturated fat: 2g; carbohydrates: 36g; fiber: 10g

Creamy Vegetable Casserole

Preparation time: 20 minutes

Servings: 2

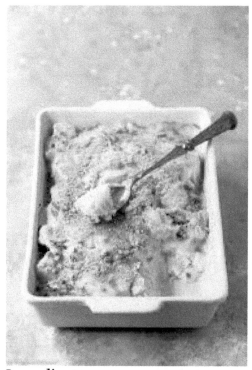

Ingredients:

Fresh rosemary (two tablespoons)

Dried basil (one teaspoon)

Dried oregano (one teaspoon)

Garlic (three cloves)

Nutritional yeast (half cup)

Salt and pepper (to taste)

Olive oil (two tablespoons)

Apple cider vinegar (two tablespoons)

Raw cashews (one cup)

Zucchini (two large)

Broccoli (one medium head)

Cauliflower (one and a half medium head)

Russet potatoes (ten medium)

Directions:

Pour boiled water over the cashews and leave to soak.

Cut up the cauliflower into small florets and boil until soft.

The potatoes in this dish will be similar to scalloped potatoes so they need to be sliced thinly. Cut carefully, but don't be too precise, just so long as they are as thin as you can get them (think really fat potato chips).

When the cauliflower is done, drain it and put it in a blender along with the drained cashews and one and a half cups of cold water. Add a good half teaspoon of salt along with the apple cider vinegar and nutritional yeast. Blend until creamy.

Wash and grate the zucchini, set aside. Cut the broccoli into small bite-sized pieces and set aside.

In a large baking dish, spread the sides and bottom with generous amounts of olive oil. Then put two layers of potatoes down so that there are no gaps to the bottom.

Pour half of the cauliflower sauce to cover and spread evenly. Add the grated zucchini and spread out to cover the sauce. Sprinkle the oregano and basil over the zucchini, then push the pieces of broccoli into the zucchini to keep the surface as even as possible.

Drizzle a little more cauliflower sauce around the broccoli pieces to fill in the gaps. Do another layer to use up the rest of the potatoes, then pour the rest of the sauce over top of that. Spread it out as evenly as possible, right to the edges to fill in all the gaps around the sides.

Sprinkle the top with a half teaspoon of black pepper and a generous pinch or two of salt. Finely chop the fresh rosemary and sprinkle that on top also. Put in the oven on 400F for forty-five minutes. It will be done when a knife pierces the potatoes without pulling them up and the top should be beautifully browned. Let it cool before serving and enjoy!

Pasta – Italian, cheesy, decadent, lasagnas; all the words that mean love and care and satisfaction. These recipes will help you share the love with your guests and remind you what true self-love is when you make them for yourself. Indulgence doesn't have to be unhealthy.

Nutrition: calories: 89; protein: 6g; total fat: 4g; saturated fat: 1g; carbohydrates: 37g; fiber: 10g

Vegan Mac and Cheese

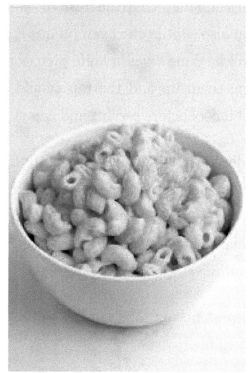

Ingredients:

Cashews (two-thirds cup raw)

Chili flakes (quarter teaspoon)

Nutritional yeast (quarter cup)

Salt and pepper (to taste)

Dry mustard powder (half teaspoon)

Onion powder (half teaspoon)

Garlic powder (half teaspoon)

Garlic (three cloves)

Russet potato (one small)

White onion (one small)

Avocado oil (one and a half tablespoons)

Broccoli (one head)

Apple cider vinegar (two teaspoons)

Macaroni (two cups)

Directions:

Peel and grate potato and grate. Finely dice the garlic.

Heat a large saucepan and oil over medium heat. Put onion and a little salt in the pot and cook until soft.

Put the potato, chili flakes and garlic along with mustard, onion and garlic powders into the pot. Stir well until their flavors release, then add one cup of water and the cashews. Keep stirring at a simmer until the potatoes are soft.

Pour entire mixture into a blender along with the apple cider vinegar and nutritional yeast, then salt and pepper. The consistency should be that of cheese sauce that is thick yet runny. If it is too thick, add more water, if it needs more salt or garlic powder, chili flakes or vinegar, do so now according to your taste.

Put the pasta on the stove in a large pot with water to cover and a little salt. In another pot, boil the broccoli in bite-sized florets until tender.

When both are ready, transfer everything into one pot and cover with the cheese sauce. Combine well, serve and enjoy!

Nutrition: calories: 263; protein: 4g; total fat: 14g; saturated fat: 2g; carbohydrates: 36g; fiber: 10g

Butternut Squash Alfredo

Ingredients:

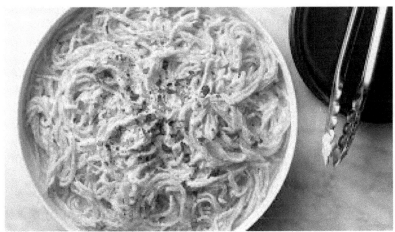

Whole grain linguine (three cups)

Vegetable broth (two cups)

Butternut Squash (three cups diced)

Salt (quarter teaspoon)

Paprika (one teaspoon)

Black pepper (half teaspoon)

Garlic (two cloves)

White onion (one medium)

Green peas (one cup)

Zucchini (one large)

Olive oil (two tablespoons)

Sage (two tablespoons fresh)

Directions:

Heat the oil in a large frypan with medium heat. While it heats, ensures the sage leaves are clean and dry, then put in the oil to fry, moving around to not burn. Pull them out and put them on a paper towel.

Into the frypan, put the peeled and diced squash along with paprika, diced onion, and black pepper. Cook until the onion is soft then add the broth and salt to taste. Bring to a boil before turning down to low heat and leaving the squash to cook through.

In another pot, cook the linguine in water with a little salt.

When the squash is tender, put it in a blender along with all the liquid and other ingredients. Blend until creamy and taste to see if more salt, pepper or spice is needed. Put it back in the frypan to keep warm on low heat.

Using a grater, grate the zucchini lengthwise to make long noodles. Make as many long ones as you can to blend in with the linguine. Add them to the sauce along with the green peas and cook in the butternut squash for five minutes.

When the pasta is done, save one cup of liquid before you drain it. Add the linguine to the pasta and stir well to coat the linguine. If the sauce is too thick, add a little of the reserved pasta water.

Serve the pasta topped with the fried sage leaves and a little blacker pepper. Enjoy!

Nutrition: calories: 32; protein: 4g; total fat: 14g; saturated fat: 2g; carbohydrates: 36g; fiber: 10g

Vegan Lasagna

Preparation time: 20 minutes

Serves: 2

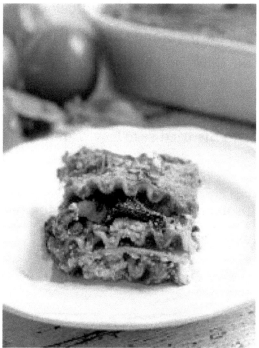

Ingredients:

Tapioca starch (four tablespoons)

Salt (half teaspoon)

Apple cider vinegar (one tablespoon)

Lemon juice (four medium lemons)

Raw cashews (one and a half cups)

Baby spinach (three cups)

Lasagna noodles (one box)

Zucchini (two medium)

Garlic powder (half teaspoon)

Dried oregano (two teaspoons)

Dried basil (two teaspoons)

Salt (one teaspoon)

Olive oil (two tablespoons)

Nutritional yeast (half cup)

Firm tofu (one pack)

Tomato puree (one mini can)

Onion powder (one tablespoon)

Garlic (six bulbs)

White onion (one medium)

Salt and pepper (to taste)

Crushed tomatoes (two cans)

Dried red lentils (one cup dried)

Directions:

Put three cups of water in a saucepan with the lentils, then bring to a boil before reducing to a simmer for around twenty minutes. Drain the lentils and set aside.

In the same saucepan, add oil and the diced onion and let cook down. When the onion is soft, add finely diced garlic, generous pinches of salt and pepper, one teaspoon each of dried oregano and basil, the two cans of crushed tomato and the one can of tomato puree. Leave to simmer for fifteen minutes, stirring every five minutes. Add the lentils to this then set aside, this is the chunky marinara.

Put half a cup of cashews into a bowl with two cups of boiled water and set aside.

Wash and slice the zucchini into lengthwise strips that are long and relatively thin then set aside.

Put one cup of cashews in a blender and pulse until crumbly. Break up the tofu and add to the blender along with the juice from one lemon, one teaspoon each of basil and oregano, the nutritional yeast, garlic powder, and a little salt. Keep pulsing until it is mostly smooth but still a little textured. Put into a bowl and set aside, this is your ricotta.

Drain the soaked cashews and put them into a clean blender with the apple cider vinegar, the juice from one lemon, tapioca starch, and a little salt. Pour in one and a half cups of water and blend until smooth. Pour this into a saucepan on medium heat and stir until it becomes stretchy then set aside. This is the cheese sauce.

In a large baking dish, place a few spoonfuls of the marinara sauce and spread it to cover the bottom and sides of the dish. Begin to layer the lasagna noodles, the ricotta, the zucchini, and the cheese sauce. Follow this with half of the spinach, more marinara, lasagna noodles, ricotta, spinach, and the cheese sauce. Keep repeating until all ingredients have been used except for a small portion of the cheese sauce.

Put into a 350F oven for one hour on the highest shelf. Remove after forty minutes and spoon the remainder of the cheese sauce over the top to resemble mozzarella blobs, then return to the oven for twenty more minutes. Let rest then serve and enjoy!

Nutrition: calories: 43; protein: 4g; total fat: 14g; saturated fat: 2g; carbohydrates: 36g; fiber: 10g

Creamy, Dreamy Dahl

Preparation time: 20 minutes

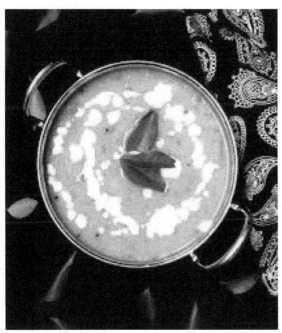

Servings: 2

Ingredients:

Fresh cilantro (small bunch)

Lemon juice (half one medium)

Red lentils (one cup dried)

Tomato (one medium)

Salt (three-quarter teaspoon)

Paprika (half teaspoon)

Ground cardamom (half teaspoon)

Turmeric (half teaspoon)

Fresh ginger (one tablespoon minced)

Garlic (four cloves)

Jalapeno (one medium)

White onion (two medium)

Cinnamon (one stick or quarter teaspoon ground)

Cumin (half teaspoon)

Coconut oil (two tablespoons)

Coconut milk (half can)

Basmati rice (one cup)

Directions:

Rinse the lentils then put in a saucepan with three cups of water and cook for twenty minutes on medium heat.

Chop the onion and finely dice the ginger, jalapeno, and garlic. Dice the tomatoes too and set aside.

Heat one tablespoon oil in a frypan on medium and put the cumin and cinnamon in the oil to release the aromas for one minute, then add the onions. Let them sweat a little before adding the garlic, ginger, and jalapeno.

In another saucepan, fill with rinsed rice, then top with water to cover. Add one tablespoon of coconut oil and the coconut milk (the liquid should be one inch above rice) and give it a quick stir. Cook on medium-high until it boils, then put the lid on and turn the heat down to medium-low and leave to simmer.

After a few minutes, put the salt, paprika, cardamom, and turmeric into the mix along with the diced tomato. If you used a cinnamon stick, pull it out now. Leave this on low to cook through.

When the lentils are done, drain them and put them back on the stove top. Scrape the tomato mixture into the lentils, along with the lemon juice and salt if needed. Mix well.

Check on the rice, and if the water has been absorbed and the rice can be easily fluffed up with a fork then it should be ready. Chop cilantro and top each serving of rice and dahl. Enjoy!

Nutrition: calories: 166; protein: 4g; total fat: 14g; saturated fat: 2g; carbohydrates: 36g; fiber: 10g

Easy Thai Coconut Curry

Preparation time: 20 minutes

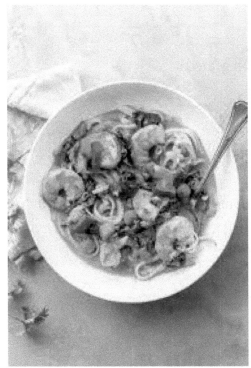

Servings: 2

Ingredients:

Jasmine rice (one cup)

Fresh basil leaves (quarter cup)

Kaffir lime leaves (three leaves)

Whole peppercorns (two tablespoons)

Snap peas (one cup)

Eggplant (one small)

Fresh ginger (one teaspoon grated)

Garlic (three cloves)

Lime juice (one medium lime)

Coconut oil (four tablespoons)

Maple syrup (one teaspoon)

Soy sauce (one tablespoon)

Firm tofu (one package)

Thai red curry paste (three tablespoons)

Coconut milk (one can)

Directions:

In a bowl, mix half the can of coconut milk with the soy sauce, maple syrup and curry paste.

Drain the tofu and cut into small cubes. Finely dice two cloves of garlic, grate the ginger and set aside. Cut the eggplant into small pieces, toss them in generous amounts of salt and set aside in a bowl.

In another saucepan, put one tablespoon coconut oil and heat on medium. Dice the last clove of garlic and put into the oil along with the rice. Stir around as the garlic cooks and the oil coats the rice. When some of the rice starts to get a little toasted, pour in water to just cover the rice and add the other half can of coconut milk along with one kefir lime leaf. Wait for it to come to a boil, then put the lid on, change heat to low and let it simmer without touching it.

Heat one tablespoon oil in a large frypan on medium and put in the tofu, cooking until all sides have been fried and are browned. Set the tofu aside.

Put in two more tablespoons of oil and put in the ginger and garlic and let fry for one minute. Rinse the salt off the eggplant, drain and put the eggplant in with the ginger and garlic.

When the eggplant gets a little soft and a little color, then add the snap peas and change heat to high. Put the curry mix into the pan and also the tofu and two of the lime leaves along with the peppercorns.

Cook for another two minutes while stirring to get everything coated and combined.

Check on the rice, it will be done when there is no liquid left and the rice can be fluffed easily with a fork. Remove the lime leaf and spoon rice onto plates.

Slice up the basil and quickly stir through the curry before spooning it over the rice. Finish with a generous squeeze of lime over everything and enjoy!

Nutrition: calories: 60; protein: 4g; total fat: 14g; saturated fat: 2g; carbohydrates: 36g; fiber: 10g

Sabrosa Spanish Paella

Preparation time: 20 minutes

Servings: 2

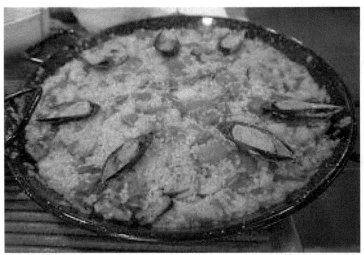

Ingredients:

Paprika (one teaspoon)

Cayenne (half teaspoon)

Saffron (one pinch)

Capers (two tablespoons)

Garlic (two cloves)

Red bell pepper (three medium)

Artichoke hearts (two small jars)

Portobello mushrooms (three cups)

Lime (one medium)

White onion (one medium)

Salt and pepper (to taste)

Olive oil (three tablespoons)

Nutritional yeast (two tablespoons)

Saffron rice (two cups)

White wine (two cups)

Vegetable stock (six cups)

Directions:

Heat a large soup pot on medium-high and put in four cups of the vegetable stock and all of the wine. Let it boil before adding all the rice, then put the lid on and allow to simmer for fifteen minutes.

Turn on the oven at 375F.

Put two red bell peppers on a baking tray and cut them in half then rub with olive oil using clean hands so they are well coated. Put in the oven cut side down and cook for twenty minutes or until they get all wrinkly and start to look a little burnt.

Get an oven-safe large frypan (if you don't have one, then use a regular frypan and get an oven dish ready for later) and heat a tablespoon of olive oil on medium before adding diced onions and one thinly sliced bell pepper.

After the onions and bell pepper become soft, put in the sliced mushrooms and leave for five more minutes.

Put into the frypan the cayenne, paprika, and saffron and stir around. Then put in the finely diced garlic, capers and artichoke hearts (without the liquid).

When the bell peppers are ready from the oven, let them cool before pulling off their skins then chop them into small slices and add to the frypan.

Drain the rice and then put in the frypan and mix well. Add generous amounts of salt and pepper at this point and taste.

If you used an oven-safe frypan, then put it into the oven. If you didn't, then transfer the pan contents into an oven dish and put that in instead.

After ten minutes, pull out the dish and add one cup of vegetable broth and mix through really well. Do this again after another ten minutes, then remove ten minutes later. The paella should have been in the oven for a total of thirty minutes.

Cut up a lime into wedges and scatter about the dish. Roughly chop fresh parsley and scatter this over top also along with the nutritional yeast. Enjoy!

ROASTS – Going vegan doesn't mean you have to give up the traditional roast, if anything, it means you get to experience unique flavors and textures that you never knew existed!

Nutrition: calories: 234; protein: 4g; total fat: 14g; saturated fat: 2g; carbohydrates: 36g; fiber: 10g

Vegan Festive Nut Roast

Preparation time: 20 minutes

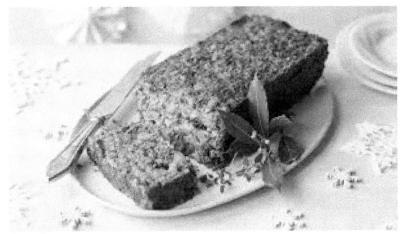

Servings: 2

Ingredients:

Paprika (two teaspoons)

Tomato puree (one teaspoon)

Miso paste (two teaspoons)

Dried rosemary (half teaspoon)

Dried sage (half teaspoon)

Dried thyme (half teaspoon)

Tahini (one tablespoon)

Dried breadcrumbs (one cup)

Chestnuts (one small can)

Raw cashews (one cup)

Carrots (one and a half cups)

Fresh rosemary (two sprigs)

Fresh thyme (two sprigs)

Butternut squash (one and a half cups)

Olive oil (one tablespoon)

Garlic (two cloves)

Onion (one medium)

Directions:

Peel and chop carrots and squash into small pieces then boil until they are very tender.

Put cashews and chestnuts into a blender and pulse until they are ground but not too fine.

Heat oil in a frypan over medium and put in chopped onion until softens. Finely dice garlic and put that in too.

Mash the carrots and squash in a bowl then add the onions and nuts. Mix very well then add every other ingredient. Well-oil a loaf sized dish and pack in firmly.

Bake at 350F covered with foil for one hour, then take off the foil and bake for another fifteen minutes.

Flip it out onto a plate and top with fresh thyme and rosemary, serve with cranberry sauce and mushroom gravy.

Nutrition: calories: 542; protein: 4g; total fat: 14g; saturated fat: 2g; carbohydrates: 36g; fiber: 10g

Roasted Vegetable Pie

Preparation time: 20 minutes

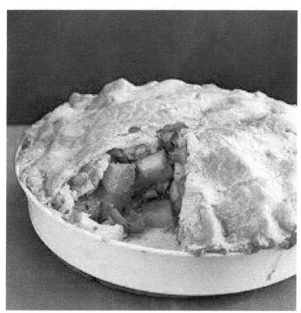

Servings: 2

Ingredients:

Vegetable suet or vegetable shortening (one cup)

White flour (one and two-thirds cup)

Salt and pepper (to taste)

Cranberry sauce (one tablespoon)

English mustard (one teaspoon)

Fresh thyme (two teaspoons)

Hazelnuts (one-third cup)

Chestnuts (one small can)

Butter beans (one can)

Dried cranberries (quarter cup)

Mushrooms (three cups)

Garlic (two cloves)

Olive oil (one tablespoon)

Leeks (one cup)

Onions (two medium)

Directions:

Heat oil in a frypan and put in the finely sliced leeks and onions. Let cook down for five minutes before adding the finely diced garlic. Put in the cranberries, drained and rinsed beans and chestnuts, chopped hazelnuts, sliced mushrooms, mustard, and thyme. Add generous pinches of salt and pepper then stir for ten minutes.

Sift flour and a half teaspoon of salt into a bowl and make a well in the middle.

Put two-thirds of a cup of water in a saucepan and bring to the boil then stir in the suet to melt.

Pour into the well of flour and gently fold the flour in until combined enough to knead. Do so for five minutes then set aside.

Oil a springform cake tin then roll out three-quarters of the pastry to lay into the tin. Spoon the cranberry sauce onto the base to cover then spoon in the vegetables.

Roll out the last quarter of the pastry and cover the vegetables. Run a knife around the edge of the lip to take off the extra pastry, then press down around the edges with a fork to pinch closed the top and base.

Drizzle and rub a tiny bit of oil over the top of the pie before you put it in the oven for one hour.

Let it sit for ten minutes before carefully lifting the sides of the cake tin and sliding the pie off the base onto a plate. Enjoy!

Nutrition: calories: 188; protein: 4g; total fat: 14g; saturated fat: 2g; carbohydrates: 36g; fiber: 10g

Epic Vegan Holiday Roast

Preparation time: 20 minutes

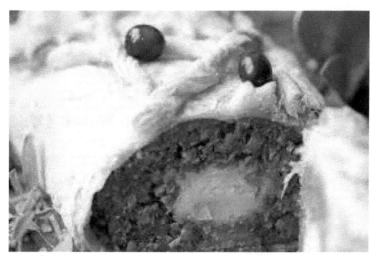

Servings: 2

Ingredients:

Salt and pepper (to taste)

Ground sage (three teaspoons)

Onion powder (three-quarter teaspoon)

Garlic powder (one teaspoon)

Soy sauce (one teaspoon)

Maple syrup (one teaspoon)

Miso paste (one tablespoon)

Olive oil (three tablespoons)

Pinto beans (half a can)

Vegetable broth (four cups)

Vital wheat gluten (two and quarter cups)

Sourdough bread (one small uncut round loaf)

Fresh parsley (half cup)

Fresh thyme (four sprigs)

Dried rosemary (one teaspoon)

Dried thyme (one tablespoon)

Mushrooms (four cups)

Garlic (five cloves)

Celery (one cup)

White onion (one large)

Barbeque sauce (two tablespoons)

Teriyaki sauce (two tablespoons)

Directions:

For the stuffing, dice the sourdough loaf into bite-sized chunks and spread over a baking tray. Bake for fifteen minutes at 350F tossing every five minutes.

Heat two tablespoons oil in a large frypan on medium and put diced onion and celery into it. When soft, add four cloves of diced garlic followed by diced mushrooms and another tablespoon of oil. Put in chopped fresh parsley with the dried rosemary, one tablespoon dried sage and the dried thyme.

When the mushrooms have cooked down, put in two cups of vegetable broth and generous sprinkles of salt and pepper. After it has simmered for five minutes, use a slotted spoon to pull out all the vegetables and put into a bowl with the bread chunks. Mix through really well then using a regular spoon, add the remaining liquid to the bread mixture until the bread has absorbed as much as it can without feeling soggy.

Oil a large baking dish and spread the contents into it before covering with aluminum wrap. Turn oven up to 375F and bake for thirty minutes covered and another twenty minutes uncovered. Set aside then turn the oven up again to 400F

In a blender put one teaspoon of sage with the onion and garlic powders. Put in one tablespoon of olive oil with the maple syrup, miso paste and one clove of whole garlic. Rinse the beans and put in along with one and a half cups of vegetable broth and one teaspoon of salt. Blend well until smooth and put into a big bowl then put in the vital wheat gluten and mix until it becomes dough-like. Use clean hands to work it (think of it like making bread) until it feels stretchy and uniforms then knead for another two minutes.

Use a rolling pin to roll it out to the size of your baking dish in a rectangle shape.

Spoon the stuffing down the center of the dough lengthwise. It should be stuffed so that when you roll it over, you have just enough dough left to pinch it together around the stuffing center. Do this the whole way down until you have a log. The stuffing should be densely packed inside so pack more in from each end if there's room.

Roll in oiled aluminum foil tightly and twist each end like a giant wrapped candy so that the roast is very tight. Put into a baking dish and pour the last half cup of broth around it like a bath and bake for ninety minutes but make sure you turn it every twenty minutes so that all sides get a chance on the bottom.

You know it's done when it feels firm to the touch much like a cooked meatloaf. Carefully unwrap the foil and put it back into the baking dish with a little drizzle of oil to stop it sticking.

Whisk together the BBQ and teriyaki sauces and pour over the roast making sure it is all coated. Put the fresh thyme sprigs on top and cook for a further ten minutes until the glaze gets sticky and darkens.

Let it rest for ten minutes then cut into rings and serve with mushroom gravy and cranberry sauce.

Nutrition: calories: 238; protein: 4g; total fat: 14g; saturated fat: 2g; carbohydrates: 36g; fiber: 10g

Chapter 9: Snack and Desserts

Cashew Raita

Servings: 21 ounces (585 g), or 12 servings

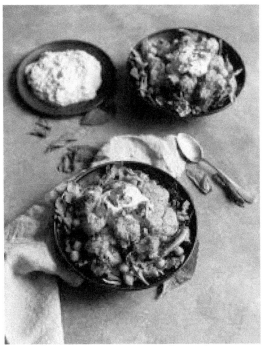

Protein content per serving: 6 g

Ingredients

For the cashew base:

1 cup (210 g) raw cashew pieces

¼ cup (60 ml) water, plus more to soak cashews, divided

¼ cup (60 ml) coconut cream

2 tablespoons (30 ml) fresh lemon juice

Protein content per serving teaspoon fine sea salt

For the raita:

1 English hothouse cucumber, cut into 6 large pieces

1 recipe cashew base

3 tablespoons (5 g) packed fresh mint leaves

3 tablespoons (11 g) packed fresh parsley

3 tablespoons (3 g) packed fresh cilantro

1 to 2 cloves garlic, grated or pressed, to taste

1 teaspoon organic lemon zest

2 teaspoons to 1 tablespoon (10 to 15 ml) fresh lemon juice

Fine sea salt

Direction

To make the cashew base: Place the cashews in a medium bowl or four-cup (940 ml) glass measuring cup. Generously cover with water. Cover with plastic wrap, or a lid, and let stand at room temperature overnight (about 8 hours) to soften the nuts.

Drain the hips (release the soaking water) and rinse quickly. Put in a high-speed food processor or mixer with a cup (60 ml) of water, coconut cream, lemon juice, and salt. To keep it soft, occasionally scrape the sides with a rubber spatula. This may take up to 10 minutes, depending on the power of the device.

Move the dispenser to a medium container covered with a lid or covered with a plastic wrap and let it sit for 24 hours at room temperature or until the smell is stained. It depends on the temperature of your location.

To make Rita: Put the cucumber in a pan and press several times until it is crushed. Add the remaining ingredients and press to mix correctly, stopping to crush the sides with a rubber floor once or twice. Adjust seasonings if necessary. Refrigerate for at least 2 hours or overnight to allow the flavors to melt. Refrigerate slowly before serving. The waste can be stored in the refrigerator for up to 4 days.

Nutrition: calories 150, fat 1, fiber 2, carbs 6, protein 5

No-Bake Choco Cashew Cheesecake

Servings: 8 to 12 servings

Protein content per serving: 9 g

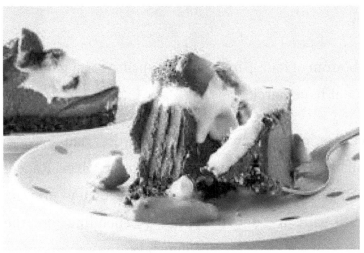

Ingredients

2 cups (280 g) raw cashews

¼ cup (60 ml) coconut cream

¼ cup (20 g) unsweetened cocoa powder

¼ cup (160 g) pure maple syrup 1 teaspoon vanilla extract

1¼ cups (125 g) walnut halves

¼ cup (89 g) chopped dates

¼ teaspoon ground cinnamon

¼ cup (30 g) almond meal, as needed

Direction

Line the bottom of four 4-inch (10 cm) spring-form pans with a parchment paper circle.

Place peanuts, coconut cream, cocoa powder, maple syrup and vanilla in a high-speed food processor or mixer. Repeat the process until it is entirely smooth, occasionally scraping the pieces with a rubber spatula. Depending on the performance of your device, this may take up to 10 minutes. Transfer the mixture to a medium bowl and set aside. Clean the food processor or blender with a paper towel.

Place the nuts, dates, and cinnamon in the same food processor or high-speed mixer. Mix and chop finely until mixed. Be careful not to over-process or make the mixture too sticky. If it is too late and the dough is too sticky, combine the almond flour. Press on the prepared pot. Put the cheese mixture in the peel and smooth from above. Place the pans in an airtight container for 3 hours and place them in the freezer to dry (this will make them less dirty), remove the cheese from the pots, and put them back in the refrigerator to prepare food.

Nutrition: calories 122, fat 1, fiber 2, carbs 6, protein 5

Cacao-Coated Almonds

Servings: 2¼ cups (320 g) almonds, or 10 servings

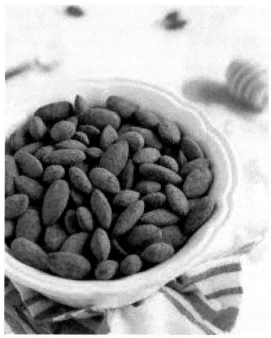

Protein content per serving: 7 grams

Ingredients

¼ cup (35 g) cacao nibs

¼ cup (38 g) light brown sugar (not packed)

1 teaspoon instant espresso powder, optional

Pinch of kosher salt

2 teaspoons cornstarch 2 teaspoons warm water

1 tablespoon (20 g) pure maple syrup

1 teaspoon pure vanilla extract

2 cups (240 g) roasted whole almonds

¼ cup (30 g) powdered sugar, optional

Direction

Preheat the oven to 325°F (170°C, or gas mark 3). Have a large rimmed baking sheet lined with parchment paper handy.

Place the cacao nibs, sugar, espresso powder, and salt in a coffee grinder. Grind to turn into a fine powder.

In a large bowl, whisk the cornstarch with the warm water until thoroughly combined. Stir the maple syrup and vanilla into the mixture. Add the almonds on top and fold until thoroughly coated.

Add the ground cacao mixture and combine until the almonds are thoroughly coated.

Place the almonds evenly on the baking sheet. Toast for 10 minutes remove from the oven and stir gently. Toast for another 5 minutes or until the coating looks mostly dry. Be careful not to allow to burn!

Let cool on the sheet. The coating will further harden once cooled. Once completely cooled, place the nuts in a bowl or Ziploc bag and dust with the sugar, shaking to coat thoroughly. Store in an airtight container in the refrigerator for up to 2 weeks.

Nutrition: calories 132, fat 1, fiber 2, carbs 6, protein 5

Smoky Bean and Tempeh Patties

Servings: 8 patties

Protein content per patty: 10 g

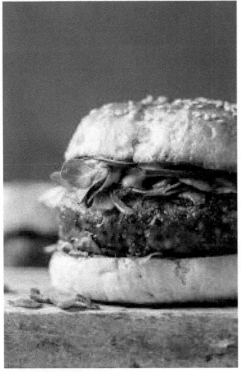

Ingredients:

1 cup (177 g) cooked cannellini beans 8 ounces (227 g) tempeh

'¼ cup (91 g) cooked bulgur

2 cloves garlic, pressed

¼ teaspoons onion powder

4 teaspoons (20 ml) liquid smoke

4 teaspoons (20 ml) vegan Worcestershire sauce

1 teaspoon smoked paprika

2 tablespoons (30 g) organic ketchup

2 tablespoons (40 g) pure maple syrup

2 tablespoons (30 ml) neutral-flavored oil

3 tablespoons (45 ml) tamari.'

¼ cup (60 g) chickpea flour

Nonstick cooking spray

Direction

Mash the beans in a large bowl: It's okay if a few small pieces of beans are left. Crumble (do not mash) the tempeh into small pieces on top. Add the bulgur and garlic. In a medium bowl, whisk together the remaining ingredients, except the flour and cooking spray. Stir into the crumbled tempeh preparation. Add the flour and mix until well combined. Chill for 1 hour before shaping into patties.

Preheat the oven to 350°F (180°C. or gas mark 4). Line a baking sheet with parchment paper. Scoop out a packed 1/3 cup (96 g) per patty, shaping into an approximately 3-inch (8 cm) circle and flattening slightly on the prepared sheet. You should get eight 3.5-inch (9 cm) patties in all. Lightly coat the top of the patties with cooking spray. Bake for 15 minutes, carefully flip, lightly coat the top of the patties with cooking spray, and bake for another 15 minutes until lightly browned and firm.

Leftovers can be stored in an airtight container in the refrigerator for up to 4 days. The patties can also be frozen, tightly wrapped in foil, for up to 3 months.

If you don't eat all the patties at once, reheat the leftovers on low heat in a skillet lightly greased with olive oil or cooking spray for about 5 minutes on each side until heated through.

Nutrition: calories 89, fat 1, fiber 2, carbs 6, protein 5

Sloppy Joe Scramble Stuffed Spuds

Servings: 6 potato halves

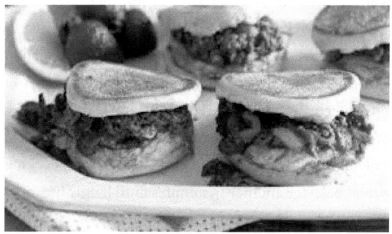

Protein content per potato half: 12 g

Ingredients

1 to 2 tablespoons (15 to 30 ml) high heat neutral-flavored oil

1 pound (454 g) extra-firm tofu, drained, pressed, and crumbled

¼ teaspoon fine sea salt

¼ teaspoon ground black pepper

¾ cup (120 g) minced onion

'¼ cup (75 g) minced bell pepper (any color)

3 cloves garlic, minced

1 tablespoon (7 g) ground cumin

2 teaspoons chili powder, or to taste

1 can (15 ounces, or 425 ml) tomato sauce

2 tablespoons (30 g) organic ketchup 1 tablespoon (15 ml) tamari

1 tablespoon (15 ml) vegan Worcestershire sauce

1 tablespoon (11 g) prepared yellow mustard

1 (4-inch or 10 cm) dill pickle, minced

¾ cup (180 ml) water

3 baked potatoes, cooled

1 tablespoon (15 ml) olive oil

Direction

Heat 1 tablespoon (15 ml) of oil in a large skillet over medium-high heat. If the skillet is not well-seasoned, add the remaining tablespoon (15 ml) of oil. Add the tofu, salt, and pepper. Cook for 8 to 10 minutes, occasionally stirring until the tofu is firm and golden. Stir in the onion, bell pepper, garlic, cumin, and chili powder. Reduce the heat to medium and cook for 3 minutes, occasionally stirring, until fragrant. Add the tomato sauce, ketchup, tamari, Worcestershire sauce, mustard, and dill pickle. Bring to a boil, and then reduce the heat to simmer. Swish the water in the tomato sauce can to clean the sides. Simmer for 30 minutes, occasionally stirring, adding the water from the tomato sauce can. As needed for the desired consistency.

Preheat the oven to broil. Cut the baked potatoes in half lengthwise. Scoop the insides from the potatoes, leaving about 1 inch (1.3 cm) of the skin intact. Brush both the insides and the outsides of the potato skins with the olive oil and place them on a baking sheet. Broil for 3 to 4 minutes until lightly browned. Remove from the oven and divide the filling evenly in the potatoes, using about ¼ cup (130 g) in each.

Nutrition: calories 150, fat 1, fiber 2, carbs 6, protein 5

Seed Crackers

Servings: About 100 crackers, or 20 servings Protein content

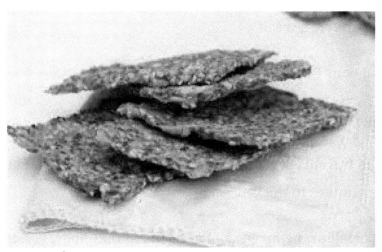

per serving: 2 g

Ingredients

3 tablespoons (36 g) white chia seeds

⅓ cup (80 ml) water, more if needed

1/3 cup (120 g) packed cooked and cooled amaranth

⅓ cup plus 2 tablespoons (75 g) whole wheat pastry flour, plus extra for rolling 3 tablespoons (30 g) shelled hemp seeds

3 tablespoons (23 g) golden roasted flaxseeds

2 tablespoons (15 g) almond meal

1½ teaspoons nutritional yeast Generous

⅓ teaspoon fine sea salt

2 tablespoons (30 ml) olive oil

Direction

Combine the chia seeds with the water in a small bowl. Let stand 2 minutes to thicken.

Add flour, flour, hemp seeds, flaxseed, almond flour, yeast, and salt. Add the thick mixture of chia and oil on top. Use a stand mixer with flat blade joints to mix perfectly. If the dough is crushed or dried, add additional water at the same time, a few drops. The mixture should be collected as a very sticky ball. Form the dough into a 5-inch (13 cm) disk. Wrap the dough tightly in a plastic wrap and refrigerate for 2 hours or overnight.

Heat the oven to 400 degrees Fahrenheit (200 degrees Celsius or gas mark 6). Draw two large baking sheets with enamel paper. Divide the dough into 4 parts.

Put a quarter of the dough on a piece of soft paper wrapped in flour, sprinkle the mixture with a little flour and cover it almost thin, almost! 4 ‹ inches (1.6 mm). Using a 2-inch (5 cm) round cutter, cut the dough into cookies and transfer it to prepared slices. Dissolve the remaining mixture until it is finished and repeat the dough for another 3 quarts. You can also wrap the remaining dough well and put it back in the refrigerator for later use for 4 days.

Cook for 8 minutes and check the softness: cracks should be browned everywhere. Some cookies are likely to bake faster than others. Take the ones that are ready and move them to a wire rack. Bake for another minute, until well cooked until lightly browned. Allow cooling on a rack before stacking in an airtight container at room temperature. You must enjoy the rest for 2 days.

Nutrition: calories 67, fat 1, fiber 2, carbs 6, protein 5

Spelt and Seed Rolls

Servings: 9 rolls

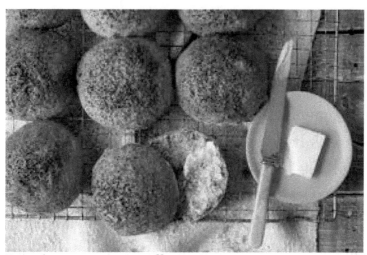

Protein content per roll: 15 g

Ingredients

1 cup (235 ml) unsweetened plain vegan milk, lukewarm

2 teaspoons apple cider vinegar

⅓ cup (120 ml) water, lukewarm

2 tablespoons (30 ml) neutral-flavored oil

2 tablespoons (40 g) agave nectar

3 cups plus scant

⅓ cup (480 g) whole spelt flour, divided

¼ cup (30 g) oat flour or finely ground oats

¼ cup (36 g) vital wheat gluten

3 tablespoons (30 g) shelled hemp seeds

3 tablespoons (25 g) sunflower seeds

2 tablespoons (15 g) golden roasted flaxseeds

2 tablespoons (24 g) chia seeds

1 tablespoon (7 g) caraway seeds or (9 g) poppy seeds

1 teaspoon fine sea salt

2 teaspoons instant yeast

Direction

Combine milk and vinegar in a measuring cup. Allow two minutes to milk. This is your "license."

Add water, oil and agave (or maple syrup or molasses) to the butter. Set aside.

In a bowl, place a 3A cup (450 g) of ground flour, oatmeal, wheat gluten, whole grains, salt, and yeast. Pour the wet ingredients over the dry ones.

Knead the dough with a stand mixer for 10 minutes until the dough becomes soft and not too dry or too sticky. If necessary, gently add 1 tablespoon (15 ml).

Cover for 75 minutes or until doubled.

Hit the dough. Place on a soft baking sheet, lightly smooth and form a circular disk approximately 10 inches (25 cm) long. Cover both sides of the disc with flour. Make 9 equal triangles from the center, similar to the buns. You can shape them or put them in round loaves.

Slowly sprinkle the extra flour and place it back on a baking sheet. Slowly lower by pressing the palm of your hand. Cover with plastic wrap. Let it grow for 25 minutes.

While the rolls rise, heat the oven to 400 degrees Fahrenheit (200 degrees Celsius, or gas mark 6). Remove the plastic wrap and do not brown or hollow it for 20 to 22 minutes or until it touches the bottom of the roll. Let cool on a rack. Store the rest in an airtight container at room temperature. Roulette is best enjoyed fresh, but it will last up to 2 days.

Nutrition: calories 159, fat 1, fiber 2, carbs 6, protein 5

Nut and Seed Sprinkles

Servings: 2 cups (225 g), or 32 servings

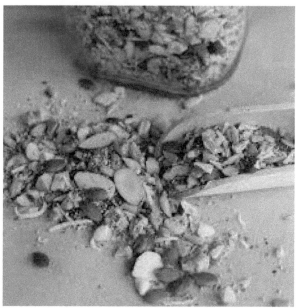

Protein content per serving: 2 g

Ingredients

1 cup (145 g) toasted whole almonds

¼ cup plus 2 tablespoons (45 g) nutritional yeast

¼ cup (40 g) shelled hemp seeds

1 teaspoon white miso, or scant ½ teaspoon fine sea salt, to taste

1 to 2 cloves garlic, grated or pressed, to taste

1½ teaspoons favorite dried herb, or a blend (dried basil, dried oregano, etc.), optional

'¼ teaspoon cayenne pepper, or to taste, optional

Direction

Place all the ingredients in a food processor. Pulse to combine until the almonds are coarsely ground to the consistency of panko bread crumbs.

Store in an airtight container in the refrigerator for up to 2 weeks.

Nutrition: calories 90, fat 1, fiber 2, carbs 6, protein 5

Almond or Cashew Biscuits

Servings: 9 biscuits

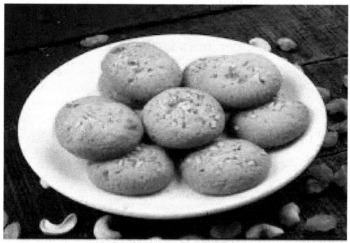

shutterstock.com • 560455729

Protein content for cookie: 15 g

Ingredients

1¼ cups (150 g) whole wheat pastry flour or (156 g) all-purpose flour

⅓ cup (47 g) toasted whole cashews or (48 g) almonds (Use unsalted.)

½ teaspoon fine sea salt

1½ teaspoons baking powder

1 tablespoon (42 g) semi-solid coconut oil (the texture of softened butter)

3 tablespoons (48 g) natural smooth cashew butter or almond butter

½ cup (120 g) blended soft silken tofu or unsweetened plain vegan yogurt

Direction

Preheat the oven to 425°F (220°C, or gas mark 7). Line a baking sheet with parch-ment paper.

Place the flour and nuts in a food processor. Pulse until the nuts are chopped: ¼ few larger pieces are okay. Add the salt and baking powder and pulse a couple of times.

Add the oil and nut butter and pulse to combine. Add the blended tofu or yogurt, and pulse until a crumbly (but not dry) dough forms. Gather the dough on a piece of parchment and pat it together to shape into a 6-inch (15 cm) square.

Cut into nine 2-inch (5 cm) square biscuits. Transfer the cookies to the prepared baking sheet. Bake for 12 to 14 minutes, or until golden brown at the edges cool on a wire rack and serve.

Nutrition: calories 100, fat 1, fiber 2, carbs 6, protein 5

Veggie Chips

Preparation time: 20 minutes

Servings: 2

Ingredients:

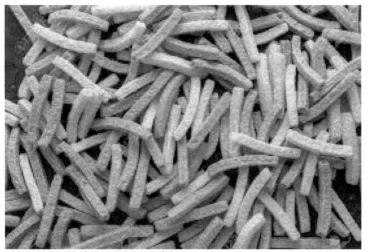

Paprika (quarter teaspoon)

Salt and pepper (to taste)

Olive oil (two teaspoons)

Sweet potato (one medium)

Directions:

Cut the sweet potato into thin slices by using a vegetable peeler. This produces even, thin, uniform slices that cook very quickly.

Put the slices into a bowl and drizzle a little oil on and toss. Repeat until every slice is coated but it shouldn't be drenched in oil.

Lay them out in a single layer with no overlapping on baking trays with baking paper.

Sprinkle with salt, pepper, and paprika to your liking.

Bake for twenty minutes at 350F, switching the trays halfway through. Be sure to keep checking them to ensure they don't overcook.

They are ready when crispy and smell amazing. Enjoy!

Nutrition: calories 99, fat 1, fiber 2, carbs 6, protein 5

Thai Vegan Rice Rolls

Preparation time: 30 minutes

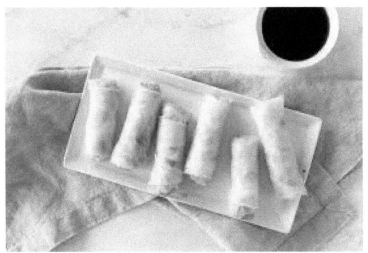

Servings: 2

Ingredients:

Rice paper rounds (three sheets)

Avocado (half one medium)

Red onion (one slice)

Carrots (two tablespoons grated)

Red bell pepper (quarter one medium)

Fresh mint leaves (six leaves)

Fresh basil leaves (six leaves)

Toasted sesame seeds (one teaspoon)

Crunchy peanut butter (one tablespoon)

Peanut oil (two tablespoons)

Soy sauce (one tablespoon)

Hot sauce (one teaspoon)

Maple syrup (one teaspoon)

Directions:

Prepare veggies and leave in individual piles on a plate. Slice avocado, bell pepper, and onion into lengthways slices. Grate the carrot, wash and de-stem the leaves.

In a bowl, put maple syrup, hot sauce, soy sauce, oil, and peanut butter and whisk together with a fork.

Run the rice paper under cool water until all parts have touched the water. Place on a clean work surface making sure they don't touch each other.

Layer the vegetables into the middle of each sheet lengthways, leaving a couple of inches away from each end. It should be a log laying in the middle of the round. Sprinkle the vegetables with the toasted sesame seeds. If the rice paper isn't 100% pliable, wait until it is. It should feel like stretchy fabric.

Fold one side over the vegetable log, then fold in both ends before rolling up like a burrito. Do this for all three, then put on a plate. Dip the roll into the peanut sauce and enjoy!

Nutrition: calories 120, fat 1, fiber 2, carbs 6, protein 5

Happy Granola Bar

Preparation time: 30 minutes

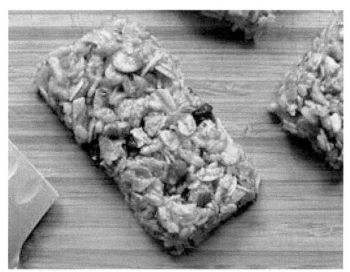

Servings: 2

Ingredients:

Chia seeds (one tablespoon)

Cinnamon (quarter teaspoon)

Desiccated coconut (quarter cup)

Almonds (three-quarter cup)

Oats (two cups)

Maple syrup (quarter cup)

Blackstrap molasses (quarter cup)

Almond butter (two-thirds cup)

Hazelnuts (quarter cup)

Cocoa powder (one teaspoon)

Directions:

Heat a saucepan over medium heat and put in the almond butter, maple syrup and molasses. Stir until the almond butter has melted down.

Take off the heat and stir in everything except the nuts.

Using a large butcher's knife, roughly chop up the almonds and hazelnuts so that they are a variety of sizes and maybe a few are left whole.

Fold the nuts through the mix and have a taste to see if it needs anything else. You could add some salt or dried berries at this point if you think it needs it.

Line a slice pan with baking paper and press the mixture into it with pressure until it is firmly packed down and relatively even in the pan.

Put in the fridge until hardened, then cut into slices and store in a container in the fridge. Enjoy!

Nutrition: calories 150, fat 1, fiber 2, carbs 6, protein 5

Peanut Butter Protein Balls

Preparation time: 30 minutes

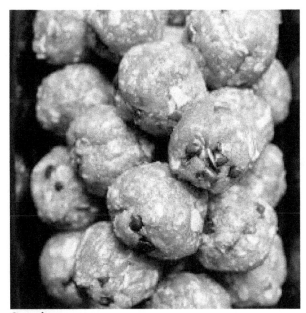

Servings: 2

Ingredients:

Almond milk (two tablespoons)

Sesame seeds (one-third cup)

Roasted sunflower seeds (one-third cup)

Vanilla extract (one teaspoon)

Maple syrup (three tablespoons)

Smooth peanut butter (half cup)

Cocoa powder (two teaspoons)

Chia seeds (one tablespoon)

Cinnamon (half teaspoon)

Chocolate vegan protein powder (half cup)

Rolled oats (one and a half cup)

Directions:

Put everything into a large bowl except for the almond milk and mix well.

Using clean hands, add the almond milk one tablespoon at a time and knead the mixture together until you get a large sticky mass.

Roll into twenty same-sized balls, tossing each one in some cocoa powder to coat. Put into a container and keep in the fridge until ready to eat. Enjoy!

Nutrition: calories 80, fat 1, fiber 2, carbs 6, protein 5

Super Seedy Cookie Bites

Preparation time: 30 minutes

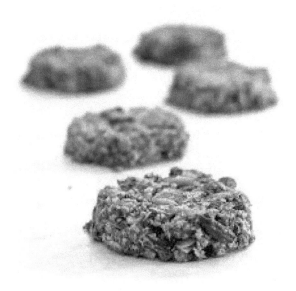

Servings: 2

Ingredients:

Shredded coconut (one cup)

Cacao nibs (two tablespoons)

Hemp hearts (three tablespoons)

Dried cranberries (quarter cup)

Raisins (quarter cup)

Pumpkin seeds (half cup)

Flaxseed meal (half cup)

Walnuts (half cup)

Medjool dates (eight)

Banana (one medium)

Directions:

Blend the dates and banana into a paste and put into a large bowl with the rest of the ingredients.

Mix together well using a little water if it needs help to combine.

Roll into twenty equal balls and lay out on a baking tray lined with baking paper. Squish each ball down slightly with your thumb to make a little cookie bite.

Cook for twenty-five minutes at 300F. Let them cool before you put in a container. Enjoy!

Nutrition: calories 87, fat 1, fiber 2, carbs 6, protein 5

Bitty Brownie Fudge Bites

Preparation time: 30 minutes

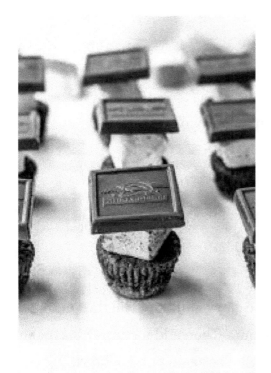

Servings: 2

Ingredients:

Cacao nibs (two tablespoons)

Cacao powder (three-quarter cups)

Salt (half teaspoon)

Dates (two and a half cups)

Coconut oil (two tablespoons)

Icing sugar (quarter cup)

Almond milk (quarter cup)

Vegan dark chocolate chips (one cup)

Raw almonds (one cup)

Raw walnuts (one and a half cups)

Directions:

In a food processor put one cup walnuts and all the almonds, pulse until a fine consistency. Then add a quarter teaspoon salt and the cacao powder. Pulse again put in a bowl.

Next, blend the dates into tiny pieces and put in a separate bowl.

Put the walnut mixture back into the processor and blend while adding tiny portions of the dates until it looks like a dough. You should be able to knead the dough and have it stick together. If it doesn't, add more dates.

Push the dough into a slice pan lined with baking paper then break up half of the remaining walnuts and sprinkle over the top along with some of the cacao nibs and press down to it's compacted and flat then put in the fridge.

Heat a saucepan over medium-low heat and put in the almond milk until it begins to simmer then take off the heat.

Add the chocolate chips and allow to melt into the milk then add a quarter teaspoon salt and the coconut oil and whisk.

Put this in the fridge for ten minutes to cool, then sift in the icing sugar and whisk it slowly to thicken the mixture, eventually whipping it like cream.

Spread the fudge over the brownie base then sprinkle with the remaining walnut pieces and cacao nibs.

Put back in the fridge to set before slicing and storing in a container either in the fridge or at room temperature. Enjoy!

Nutrition: calories 100, fat 1, fiber 2, carbs 6, protein 5

Healthy Salted Caramel Bar

Preparation time: 30 minutes

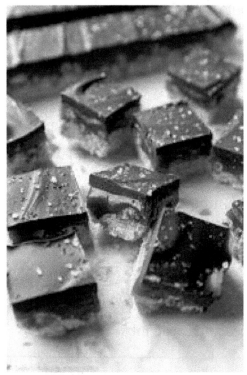

Servings: 2

Ingredients:

Almond milk (two tablespoons)

Maple syrup (two tablespoons)

Vanilla extract (one and quarter teaspoons)

Cocoa powder (third cup)

Coconut oil (half cup)

Salt (quarter teaspoon)

Cashew butter (quarter cup)

Almond milk (two teaspoons)

Medjool dates (one and a half cup)

Shredded coconut (half cup)

Almond flour (one cup)

Directions:

In a food processor put coconut oil, four dates, shredded coconut, and almond flour and blend. Evenly push it into a baking paper lined slice pan and put it in the freezer.

Next, using the processor again, put the rest of the dates along with the salt, one teaspoon vanilla, almond milk, and cashew butter. Blend until smooth and add to the top of the slice pan and put back in the freezer.

Heat the coconut oil in a saucepan on low and mix in the cocoa powder, quarter teaspoon vanilla with the maple syrup and stir until a consistent texture.

Pour this over the slice pan once it has cooled off, top with a sprinkling of shredded coconut, and put it in the fridge for two hours. Slice and enjoy!

Nutrition: calories 76, fat 1, fiber 9, carbs 6, protein 5

Chocolate Avocado Pudding

Preparation time: 30 minutes

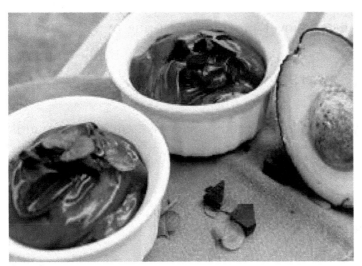

Servings: 2

Ingredients:

Maple syrup (quarter cup)

Salt (pinch)

Vanilla extract (half teaspoon)

Almond milk (four tablespoons)

Cocoa powder (quarter cup)

Vegan dark chocolate chips (quarter cup)

Ripe avocados (two medium)

Directions:

Heat a saucepan over medium and bring to a simmer the maple syrup and the almond milk. Take off the heat and stir in the chocolate chips to melt then set aside to cool.

Put everything else in a food processor then add in the milk mixture and blend until 100% smooth.

Spoon into individual portion containers, cover and put in the fridge until set. Enjoy!

Nutrition: calories 65, fat 1, fiber 2, carbs 4, protein 5

Decadent Chocolate Cake

Preparation time: 30 minutes

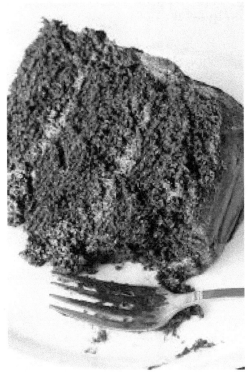

Servings: 2

Ingredients:

Vanilla extract (two teaspoons)

Almond butter (two tablespoons)

Almond milk (two and quarter cups)

Icing sugar (two and a half cups)

Cocoa powder (one and quarter cups)

Dark chocolate vegan chips (quarter cups)

Apple cider vinegar (two teaspoons)

Vegan butter (three-quarter cup)

Applesauce (one cup)

Coconut oil (half cup)

Salt (quarter cup)

Baking powder (half teaspoon)

Baking soda (three teaspoons)

Raw cane sugar (one and a half cups)

Flour (two and a half cups)

Directions:

Get a large bowl and sift into it the flour, baking powder, baking soda, sugar, salt and a three-quarter cup of cocoa and stir through.

In a saucepan on low heat melt the coconut oil quickly then take off the heat. Put in the vinegar, one teaspoon vanilla, applesauce and two cups of the milk then mix well.

Put everything together and mix with an electric beater until it's really smooth.

Pour into two 8-inch cake pans lined with baking paper and bake for forty-five minutes at 350F. Check by inserting a knife to the center at an angle, if the knife is clean when you remove it, then it is cooked through. Leave to cool.

In a clean saucepan, melt together the vegan butter and chocolate chips on low heat while stirring.

In a bowl, sift in the rest of the cocoa powder with the icing sugar, one teaspoon vanilla, almond butter and the rest of the almond milk. Pour in the chocolate butter and mix with an electric beater until thick and creamy.

Slice the very top off of one cake to make it flat and spoon some frosting on top. Spread it around before adding the second cake. Ice the entire double-stacked cake with the rest of the icing, starting with the top and then moving the icing down around the edges.

Sprinkle the top with whatever you like! Chocolate shavings or shredded coconut, chopped nuts or berries. Enjoy!

Nutrition: calories 54, fat 1, fiber 2, carbs 6, protein 5

Vegan Cheesecake with Blueberries

Preparation time: 30 minutes

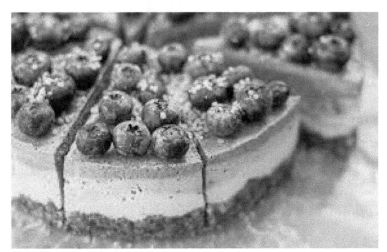

Servings: 2

Ingredients:

Chia seeds (one tablespoon)

Lemon juice (three tablespoons)

Blueberries (one cup fresh or frozen)

Freeze-dried blueberries (quarter cup)

Vanilla extract (one tablespoon)

Maple syrup (third cup)

Coconut oil (quarter cup plus two tablespoons)

Coconut milk (half cup)

Raw cashews (two cups)

Salt (quarter teaspoon)

Cinnamon (one teaspoon)

Dates (two)

Almond flour (half cup)

Raw pecans (half cup)

Directions:

Soak the cashews in boiled water an hour before starting and set aside.

In a food processor, put the pecans along with the pitted dates, two tablespoons coconut oil, almond flour, salt, and cinnamon and blend to a slightly choppy, nutty dough.

Press into the base of a six-inch cake tin that is either a well-oiled springform tin or a baking paper lined regular cake tin that will enable the cheesecake to be lifted out when done.

In the same processor, put the soaked and drained cashews with the coconut milk, maple syrup, remaining coconut oil, two tablespoons of lemon juice and vanilla. Blend until creamy, adding a little more coconut milk if necessary. If the filling needs more of anything, now is the time to add it; either vanilla, lemon, salt or syrup.

Pour two thirds over the nut base and drop the pan on the counter a few times to let it settle before placing in the freezer.

Put the freeze-dried berries into the rest of the mixture and blend to a beautiful purple filling and pour over the top of the cheesecake, dropping as before to settle.

In a blender, put the chia seeds, a tablespoon of lemon and whole blueberries. Blend and pour over the top before putting back into the freezer for three hours.

Remove from the cake tin before serving and slice with a warm knife. Enjoy!

Nutrition: calories 76, fat 8, fiber 2, carbs 6, protein 5

Do the Cocoa Shake

Servings: 4 servings, 1 cup (235 ml) per serving

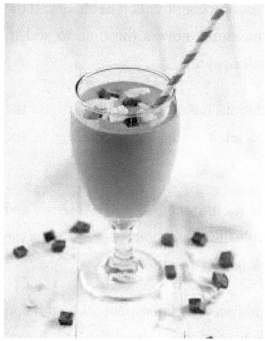

Protein content per serving: 11 g

Ingredients

12 ounces (340 g) soft silken tofu

1 (355 ml) unsweetened plain or vanilla vegan milk of choice

¼ cup (80 g) agave nectar or pure maple syrup, adjust to taste

¼ cup (64 g) natural creamy peanut or almond butter, slightly salted is fine

¼ cup (20 g) unsweetened cocoa powder

1 teaspoon pure vanilla extract

2 tablespoons (20 g) hemp powder, optional

1 frozen banana (peeled before freezing in a plastic sandwich bag), optional

Ice cubes, optional

Direction

Combine all the ingredients in a blender and blend until perfectly smooth. Add hemp powder for an extra boost of protein, a sliced frozen banana for a thicker and fruitier shake, or ice cubes for a colder, thicker shake without any added flavor.

Serve immediately or refrigerate for later use: be sure to only add the ice cubes upon serving, if storing for later. Stir well or blend again if adding ice cubes.

Nutrition: calories 150, fat 1, fiber 9, carbs 6, protein 5

Smoky Bean and Tempeh Patties

Servings: 8 patties

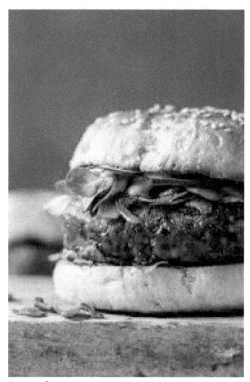

Protein content per patty: 10 g

Ingredients:

1 cup (177 g) cooked cannellini beans 8 ounces (227 g) tempeh

'¼ cup (91 g) cooked bulgur

2 cloves garlic, pressed

¼ teaspoons onion powder

4 teaspoons (20 ml) liquid smoke

4 teaspoons (20 ml) vegan Worcestershire sauce

1 teaspoon smoked paprika

2 tablespoons (30 g) organic ketchup

2 tablespoons (40 g) pure maple syrup

2 tablespoons (30 ml) neutral-flavored oil

3 tablespoons (45 ml) tamari.'

¼ cup (60 g) chickpea flour

Nonstick cooking spray

Direction

Mash the beans in a large bowl: It's okay if a few small pieces of beans are left. Crumble (do not mash) the tempeh into small pieces on top. Add the bulgur and garlic. In a medium bowl, whisk together the remaining ingredients, except the flour and cooking spray. Stir into the crumbled tempeh preparation. Add the flour and mix until well combined. Chill for 1 hour before shaping into patties.

Preheat the oven to 350°F (180°C. or gas mark 4). Line a baking sheet with parchment paper. Scoop out a packed 1/3 cup (96 g) per patty, shaping into an approximately 3-inch (8 cm) circle and flattening slightly on the prepared sheet. You should get eight 3.5-inch (9 cm) patties in all. Lightly coat the top of the patties with cooking spray. Bake for 15 minutes, carefully flip, lightly coat the top of the patties with cooking spray, and bake for another 15 minutes until lightly browned and firm.

Leftovers can be stored in an airtight container in the refrigerator for up to 4 days. The patties can also be frozen, tightly wrapped in foil, for up to 3 months.

If you don't eat all the patties at once, reheat the leftovers on low heat in a skillet lightly greased with olive oil or cooking spray for about 5 minutes on each side until heated through.

Nutrition: calories 130, fat 1, fiber 2, carbs 6, protein 8

Spelt and Seed Rolls

Servings: 9 rolls

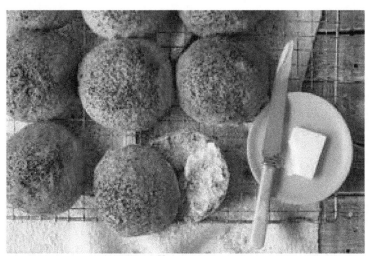

Protein content per roll: 15 g

Ingredients

1 cup (235 ml) unsweetened plain vegan milk, lukewarm

2 teaspoons apple cider vinegar

⅓ cup (120 ml) water, lukewarm

2 tablespoons (30 ml) neutral-flavored oil

2 tablespoons (40 g) agave nectar

3 cups plus scant

⅓ cup (480 g) whole spelt flour, divided

¼ cup (30 g) oat flour or finely ground oats

¼ cup (36 g) vital wheat gluten

3 tablespoons (30 g) shelled hemp seeds

3 tablespoons (25 g) sunflower seeds

2 tablespoons (15 g) golden roasted flaxseeds

2 tablespoons (24 g) chia seeds

1 tablespoon (7 g) caraway seeds or (9 g) poppy seeds

1 teaspoon fine sea salt

2 teaspoons instant yeast

Direction

Combine milk and vinegar in a measuring cup. Allow two minutes to milk. This is your "license."

Add water, oil and agave (or maple syrup or molasses) to the butter. Set aside.

In a bowl, place a 3A cup (450 g) of ground flour, oatmeal, wheat gluten, whole grains, salt, and yeast. Pour the wet ingredients over the dry ones.

Knead the dough with a stand mixer for 10 minutes until the dough becomes soft and not too dry or too sticky. If necessary, gently add 1 tablespoon (15 ml).

Cover for 75 minutes or until doubled.

Hit the dough. Place on a soft baking sheet, lightly smooth and form a circular disk approximately 10 inches (25 cm) long. Cover both sides of the disc with flour. Make 9 equal triangles from the center, similar to the buns. You can shape them or put them in round loaves.

Slowly sprinkle the extra flour and place it back on a baking sheet. Slowly lower by pressing the palm of your hand. Cover with plastic wrap. Let it grow for 25 minutes.

While the rolls rise, heat the oven to 400 degrees Fahrenheit (200 degrees Celsius, or gas mark 6). Remove the plastic wrap and do not brown or hollow it for 20 to 22 minutes or until it touches the bottom of the roll. Let cool on a rack. Store the rest in an airtight container at room temperature. Roulette is best enjoyed fresh, but it will last up to 2 days.

Nutrition: calories 56, fat 1, fiber 2, carbs 4, protein 5

Nut and Seed Sprinkles

Servings: 2 cups (225 g), or 32 servings

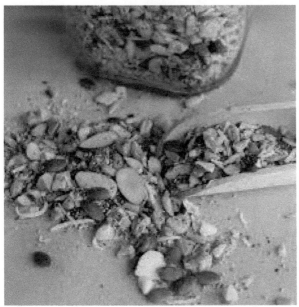

Protein content per serving: 2 g

Ingredients

1 cup (145 g) toasted whole almonds

¼ cup plus 2 tablespoons (45 g) nutritional yeast

¼ cup (40 g) shelled hemp seeds

1 teaspoon white miso, or scant ½ teaspoon fine sea salt, to taste

1 to 2 cloves garlic, grated or pressed, to taste

1½ teaspoons favorite dried herb, or a blend (dried basil, dried oregano, etc.), optional

'¼ teaspoon cayenne pepper, or to taste, optional

Direction

Place all the ingredients in a food processor. Pulse to combine until the almonds are coarsely ground to the consistency of panko bread crumbs.

Store in an airtight container in the refrigerator for up to 2 weeks.

Nutrition: calories 65, fat 1, fiber 2, carbs 6, protein 5

Almond or Cashew Biscuits

Servings: 9 biscuits

Protein content for cookie: 15 g

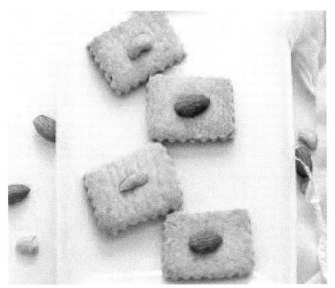

Ingredients

1¼ cups (150 g) whole wheat pastry flour or (156 g) all-purpose flour

⅓ cup (47 g) toasted whole cashews or (48 g) almonds (Use unsalted.)

½ teaspoon fine sea salt

1½ teaspoons baking powder

1 tablespoon (42 g) semi-solid coconut oil (the texture of softened butter)

3 tablespoons (48 g) natural smooth cashew butter or almond butter

½ cup (120 g) blended soft silken tofu or unsweetened plain vegan yogurt

Direction

Preheat the oven to 425°F (220°C, or gas mark 7). Line a baking sheet with parch-ment paper.

Place the flour and nuts in a food processor. Pulse until the nuts are chopped: ¼ few larger pieces are okay. Add the salt and baking powder and pulse a couple of times.

Add the oil and nut butter and pulse to combine. Add the blended tofu or yogurt, and pulse until a crumbly (but not dry) dough forms. Gather the dough on a piece of parchment and pat it together to shape into a 6-inch (15 cm) square.

Cut into nine 2-inch (5 cm) square biscuits. Transfer the cookies to the prepared baking sheet. Bake for 12 to 14 minutes, or until golden brown at the edges cool on a wire rack and serve.

Nutrition: calories 50, fat 1, fiber 2, carbs 5, protein 5

Mushroom Cashew Mini Pies

Servings: 24 mini pies

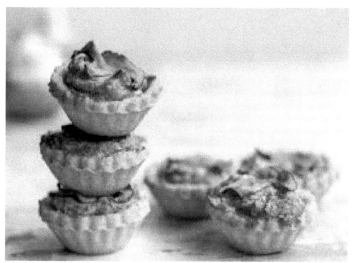

Protein content for cake: 2 g

Ingredients

For the filling:

1 scant cup (210 g) Creamy Cashew Baking Spread

1/3 cup (80 g) minced rehydrated dried mushrooms of choice

¼ cup (15 g) chopped fresh parsley

2 tablespoons (20 g) minced red onion

2 tablespoons (15 g) nutritional yeast

2 cloves garlic, grated or pressed

¼ teaspoon fine sea salt

¼ teaspoon ground nutmeg Ground black or white pepper

For the crusts:

Nonstick cooking spray

1¼ cups (150 g) whole wheat pastry flour

¼ cup (40 g) hemp powder

Scant ½ teaspoon fine sea salt

2 tablespoons (32 g) cashew butter

2 tablespoons (30 ml) neutral-flavored oil

¼ cup plus 2 tablespoons (90 ml) cold unsweetened plain vegan milk, as needed

Direction

To make the filling: In a medium bowl, combine all the ingredients with a spoon until thoroughly mixed. Set aside while preparing the crusts.

To make the crusts: Preheat the oven to 350°F (180°C, or gas mark 4). Lightly coat a 24-cup mini muffin pan with cooking spray. Place the flour, hemp powder, and salt in a large bowl. In a small bowl, stir to combine the cashew butter and oil. Using a fork, cut the cashew butter mixture into the flour mixture. Add ¼ cup (60 ml) of the milk, stirring until crumbs form, adding an extra table-spoon (15 ml) at a time if needed. The crumbs of dough should stick together easily when pinched and be neither too dry, nor too wet.

Place a generous 1¼ teaspoons of crumbs in each muffin cup, pressing down to fit the bottom and sides of the bowl. Add 2 generous teaspoons of filling the per crust, smoothing out the tops. Bake for 22 minutes or until the tops are firm and light golden brown. Remove from the pan, transfer to a wire rack, and serve warm or at room temperature. Leftovers can be stored in an airtight container in the refrigerator for up to 2 days and reheated in a 325°F (170°C, or gas mark 3) oven until warm, about 15 minutes.

Nutrition: calories 150, fat 1, fiber 2, carbs 6, protein 5

Tempeh Koftas with Cashew Dip

Servings: 20 koftas. plus 1 scant cup (230 g) dip

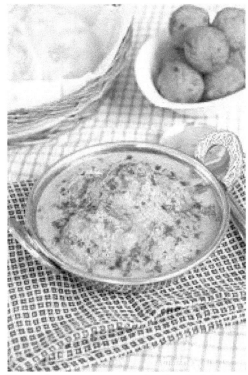

Protein content per kofta (with sauce): 6 g

For the simple cashew dip:

¾ cup (180 g) cashew base

1½ tablespoons (6 g) packed minced fresh parsley

1 ¼ tablespoon (23 ml) fresh lemon juice

1½ tablespoons (24 g) tahini

1 to 2 cloves garlic, grated or pressed, to taste

Salt and pepper

For the koftas:

Nonstick cooking spray

1 cup (177 g) cannellini beans or 1 cup (171 g) black-eyed peas

8 ounces (227 g) tempeh

¾ cup (40 g) minced red onion

¾ cup (16 g) packed flat-leaf parsley, minced

2 tablespoons (30 ml) neutral-flavored oil, plus extra for brushing

1 tablespoon (15 g) harissa paste

3 large cloves garlic, grated or pressed

1½ teaspoons ground coriander

1 teaspoon ground cumin

teaspoon fine sea salt

¼ teaspoon ground cinnamon

¼ teaspoon ground allspice

¼ teaspoon ground nutmeg

2 tablespoons (15 g) whole wheat pastry flour or (16 g) all-purpose flour

2 tablespoons (30 ml) fresh lemon juice, optional

Olive oil, for brushing

Direction

To make the cuttings: 20 cups Cover a small roll of muffins with 24 cups of spray oil.

Grate beans or peas in a large bowl: if there are only a few beans left, that's fine. Chop the top into small pieces (do not crush). Add onions, parsley, oil. Cover the harissa paste, garlic, coriander, cumin, salt, cinnamon, spice flour, nutmeg, and flour.

Stir to combine. If the mixture is dry and does not come together, add the lemon juice and stir to combine. Place a tablespoon of the round and round mixture (approximately 25 grams) on a ball and place it in a muffin pan. Repeat with the remaining bushes. Cover with a loose plastic wrap and refrigerate for 1 hour.

Heat the oven to 350 degrees F (180 degrees Celsius or gas mark 4).

Gently brush each bush with oil. Bake for 15 minutes, turn gently (fins will be brittle) and brush lightly with oil again. Bake for another 10 minutes or until golden brown.

Leave it on the muffin hook for 10 minutes before serving, as the soles of the foot will be brittle just outside the stove. Serve with drunken almonds. The buttercups are also delicious.

For dehydration: combine all ingredients in a food processor to combine. Occasionally, stop jamming the sides with a rubber spatula. Cover and keep for at least 1 hour in the refrigerator until ready to serve. Remnants can be stored in a refrigerated container for up to 3 days. The sink thickens after more than 24 hours after freezing. Use it, as it spreads on bread or adds more lemon juice to taste.

Nutrition: calories 123, fat 1, fiber 8, carbs 6, protein 5

Seed and Nut Ice Cream

Servings: 1 quart (950 ml), or 8 servings

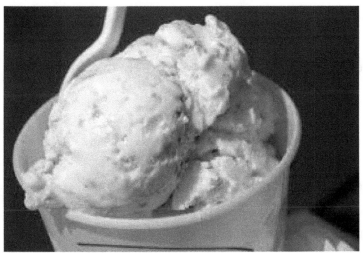

Protein content per serving: 9 g

Ingredients

For the nuts:

1 1/3 tablespoons (30 g) pure maple syrup

1/3 teaspoon ground cinnamon

¼ teaspoon ground nutmeg

¼ teaspoon fine sea salt

1/3 cup (50 g) walnut or pecan halves

For the ice cream:

1/3 cup (128 g) tahini

⅓ cup (128 g) natural creamy cashew butter or peanut butter

12 ounces (340 g) soft silken tofu, or ugly or vanilla vegan yogurt

1/3 cup plus 2 tablespoons (200 g) agave nectar

¼ cup (60 ml) full-fat coconut milk

1/3 teaspoon ginger powder

1/3 teaspoon ground cinnamon

1½ teaspoons pure vanilla extract

Direction

To make the nuts: Preheat the oven to 325°F (170°C, or gas mark 3).

In a medium bowl, mix maple syrup, cinnamon, nutmeg, and salt. Add half of the nut or walnut and stir to foam. Place on a baking sheet with oil on a nonstick baking sheet and bake for 8 minutes. Stir for another 4 to 6 minutes to heat and dry and be careful not to dry. Before crushing, remove from oven and allow to cool completely. Set aside.

To make ice cream: Freeze your ice cream tub for at least 24 hours.

Put all the ingredients in the blender and mix until smooth. Try a little of the mixture to make sure it is sweet and sweet enough to your liking and, if desired, add 1 tablespoon (15 ml) at a time to the sweetener. If you make adjustments, mix again.

Transfer the mixture to the ice cream machine and follow the ice cream preparation Direction. Add chopped nuts during the last 5 minutes of shake. Transfer to a container and refrigerate for 2 hours. After more than a couple of hours, the ice cream does not want to be poured directly from the freezer, so let it sit for 15 minutes at room temperature.

Nutrition: calories 150, fat 1, fiber 2, carbs 5, protein 5

Cheesy Popcorn

Ingredients:

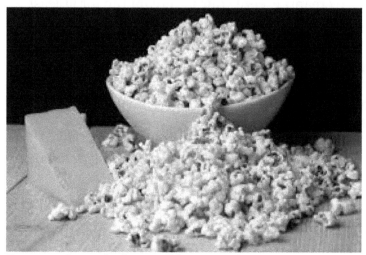

Popcorn kernels (two tablespoons)

Grapeseed oil (one tablespoon)

Coconut oil (one tablespoon)

Pink or sea salt (to taste)

Nutritional yeast (one tablespoon)

Black pepper (to taste)

DIRECTION:

Heat coconut oil in a saucepan over medium heat. Put in the popcorn, apply the lid and shake the pot side to side to coat the kernels in the oil. Leave pot still until you hear the popcorn start to pop. Shake the pot periodically to ensure no popcorn sticks to the bottom and the un-popped kernels find their way to the bottom.

When the popping begins to slow, get your bowl ready and tip the popcorn into it when the popping has practically stopped.

Drizzle the popcorn with the grapeseed oil and toss through, then generously apply salt to your liking, top with the nutritional yeast. Give it a good shake again so the yeast has a chance to stick to the oil, then sprinkle a little black pepper over top. Enjoy!

Nutrition: calories 170, fat 1, fiber 2, carbs 6, protein 5

Chapter 10: A 21-Day Vegan Meal Plan and Shopping List

DAY	BREAKFAST	LUNCH/DINNER	SNACK/DESSERT
1.	Green Kickstart Smoothie	Herby Giant Couscous with Asparagus and Lemon	Cashew Raita
2.	Warm Quinoa Breakfast Bowl	Veggieful' Chili	Nut and Seed Sprinkles
3.	Banana Bread Rice Pudding	Red Curry Lentils	Almond or Cashew Biscuits
4.	Apple and cinnamon oatmeal	Black-Bean Veggie Burritos	Veggie Chips
5.	Spiced orange breakfast couscous	Baked Red Bell Peppers	Thai Vegan Rice Rolls

6.	Breakfast parfaits	Quick Quinoa Casserole	Happy Granola Bar
7.	Sweet potato and kale hash	Mexican Casserole	Peanut Butter Protein Balls
8.	Delicious Oat Meal	Mushroom Ragout	Super Seedy Cookie Bites
9.	Breakfast Cherry Delight	Pumpkin Pilaf	Bitty Brownie Fudge Bites
10.	Crazy Maple and Pear Breakfast	Baked Root Veg with Chili	Healthy Salted Caramel Bar
11.	Hearty French Toast Bowls	Autumn Stuffed Enchiladas	Chocolate Avocado Pudding
12.	Tofu Burrito	Creamy Vegetable Casserole	Decadent Chocolate Cake
13.	Tasty Mexican Breakfast	Vegan Mac and Cheese	Vegan Cheesecake

			with Blueberries
14.	Green Kickstart Smoothie	Butternut Squash Alfredo	Do the Cocoa Shake
15.	Warm Quinoa Breakfast Bowl	Vegan Lasagna	Smoky Bean and Tempeh Patties
16.	Banana Bread Rice Pudding	Creamy, Dreamy Dahl	Spelt and Seed Rolls
17.	Apple and cinnamon oatmeal	Easy Thai Coconut Curry	Nut and Seed Sprinkles
18.	Spiced orange breakfast couscous	Sabrosa Spanish Paella	Almond or Cashew Biscuits
19.	Breakfast parfaits	Vegan Festive Nut Roast	Mushroom Cashew Mini Pies

20.	Sweet potato and kale hash	Roasted Vegetable Pie	Tempeh Koftas with Cashew Dip
21.	Hearty French Toast Bowls	Epic Vegan Holiday Roast	Seed and Nut Ice Cream

Shopping List

Fruit & veg

Asparagus spears

Avocados

Baby carrots (e.g. Chantenay)

Handful baby spinach

large carrot small baby carrots

Cherry tomatoes

Curly kale

Fresh basil

Fresh coriander

Lemons

Lime

Mixed mushrooms

Onions

Baking potatoes

Red onions

Romano peppers

Shallots mon

Spring onions

Sweet potato

Tins & dried goods

Borlotti beans (tinned)

Brazil nuts

Tin cannellini beans

Cashew nuts

Tin chickpeas

Tin chopped tomatoes

Gnocchi (ready-made, check it is vegan)

Tin green or brown lentils

Microwave packet brown basmati rice

Passata

Roasted red pepper (from a jar)

Spelt spaghetti (or normal wheat spaghetti would be fine too)

Sultanas Tue

Tinned black beans

Whole-wheat giant couscous

Alcohol

White wine (check it is vegan -you can buy a 250ml bottle and freeze the rest for next time)

Bakery

Tortilla wraps (or 4 small wraps) Wed

Chiller Cabinet

Coconut yoghurt

Dairy-free cream (soya or oat cream)

Vegan parmesan-style 'cheese'

Vegan sausages

Freezer

Peas (fresh or frozen)

Vegetables and pulses (e.g. bag frozen Chickpea & Spinach mix with lentils and spinach)

PLANT-BASED DIET COOKBOOK FOR BEGINNERS

Chapter 11: The importance of plant-based food for the athlete for a strong and healthy body.

Protein is a macronutrient and a very important constituent of a diet weather you are looking to build muscle or not, as:

It is a constituent of all body cells. As a matter of fact, nails and hair are mostly made of protein.

Protein is required to repair and build tissue.

Hormones, enzymes, and many other important body chemicals are made up of protein.

It is a vital building block of cartilage, muscles, bones, skin, and blood.

Our bodies do not stock up on protein like they do carbohydrates and fats, hence it has no reserve to draw from when the dietary requirement is not being met.

Benefits of a Protein-Enriched Diet

Consuming high-protein foods has many benefits, including:

- Speedy revitalization after work outs
- Reducing muscle loss

- Building muscle mass

- Helping you maintain a healthy weight

- Reducing appetite

Sources of plant protein include: Legumes such as peas, black beans, soy beans – popular forms include edamame, tempeh, soy milk and tofu, and chickpeas - grains such as corn, bulgur, brown rice, barley, and wheat-often eaten as seitan and whole-wheat bread; and seeds and nuts, such as sunflower seeds hemp, flax and almonds, peanuts etc.

Quinoa and soy beans are complete proteins since they both have all the important amino acids in quantities that meet human demands.

Plant-based diets are becoming widely popular, and more and more people are switching to plant-based diets for a variety of reasons. Diets that are based on consumption of plant foods and are rich in beans, nuts, seeds, fruit and vegetables, whole grains, and cereal-based foods can provide all the nutrients needed for good health and offer affordable, tasty and nutritious alternatives to meat-based diets.

Scientific research provides evidence that switching to plant-based diets helps control, reduce and even reverse various chronic diseases. Analysis of the question given in the book called The China Study highlights the fact that plant-based diets that are also low in saturated fat, can help control weight and may reduce the risk of type 2 diabetes, cardiovascular and heart diseases, some types of cancer and other significant illnesses. There are also reports of having more energy, reduced inflammation, bigger fitness payoffs, and better overall health outcomes after switching to a plant-based diet.

However, as with any diet, this diet will require detailed planning and if thought through well, it can provide and support healthy living at every age and stage of life. Here are several steps that can help with switching and maintaining the plant-based diet:

•	Start slowly by selecting a few easy to prepare plant-based meals that you enjoy and use them throughout the week. Once you try that and are satisfied with the outcome, you can expand further adding more dishes.

•	Slowly lower the consumption of meat and processed foods. Start by reducing the proportion of animal-sourced foods in your every meal. Eat more salads, vegetables, and fruits. Then lower the consumption of dairy products if you plan on going 100% vegan and start replacing with plant-based alternatives.

- Once you are confident enough and satisfied with the results, you can try making one complete meal in your daily ration fully vegan.

- Next, you need to watch your protein intake. While our body needs to get 1 gram per 1 kg of weight every day, overconsumption of protein is not necessary and can even be harmful. And since plants have more than enough proteins, you might want to start watching them.

- In general, it's best to stick to whole, intact foods as much as possible. There are lots of right products on the market today to stay healthy and adhere to the plant-based path.

Energy & Performance; Protein and Recovery

Plant-based diets are also becoming popular and widely accepted by professional athletes. There are several reasons for that.

Even athletes are prone to the risk of cardiovascular and heart diseases, and a plant-based diet is right in keeping heart healthy and problem-free, lowering blood pressure and cholesterol level. Meat consumption and cholesterol from it can cause inflammation, which can result in lower athletic performance and slower recovery. Plant-based diet shows have anti-inflammatory effect. It also improves blood thickness, which results in more oxygen reaching muscles, which in turn improves athletic performance. It also makes arteries more flexible and more prominent in diameter resulting in better blood flow. One study shows that even one high-fat meal worsens arterial function for several hours. People that follow the plant-based diet get more antioxidants, which help in neutralizing free radicals that cause muscle fatigue, impaired recovery, and reduced athletic performance. A plant-based diet can reduce body fat, which can increase aerobic capacity that is vital to exercising through using more oxygen to fuel muscles. Studies indicate that athletes following the plant-based diet have increased maximum level of oxygen they can use while applying resulting in better endurance.

Muscle Protein Synthesis

Muscle Protein Synthesis is a process that is vital to the human body. Proteins are the compounds that are built from amino acids, which appear to be the building material for the creation of tissues in the human body, and Muscle Protein Synthesis is a naturally occurring process in which protein is produced to assist with the growth, repair and overall maintenance of human skeletal muscles. It is an opposing process to the Muscle Protein Breakdown, during which protein is being lost after exercising.

Muscle Protein Synthesis also closely correlates with exercising that muscles receive, as muscle growth can be achieved only through regular training and proper protein intake. Human skeletal muscles will not grow or get stronger without exercising, and in such case, Muscle Protein Synthesis will not be of any help and will only be doing ongoing repairs and maintenance of existing muscle tissues.

To accelerate muscle growth, improve athletic performance, endurance and recovery you will need to learn how to stimulate Muscle Protein Synthesis through the combination of exercise and appropriate diet.

There is a relationship between Muscle Protein Synthesis and Muscle Protein Breakdown and is called Protein Balance. To stimulate the growth of muscles a person needs to unsettle that protein balance, and to do that all that needs to be done is train hard, and the greater the intensity of exercising, the higher the Muscle Protein Synthesis. The correlation between diet and Muscle Protein Synthesis is not as straightforward as applying. Even if protein intake rises, Muscle Protein Synthesis increases for a short period. It is because body can only utilize a certain amount of amino acids that it receives, and everything above that certain amount will get broken down and excreted by the liver.

Macros & Micros

Macronutrients or macros and micronutrients or micros are molecules that the human body needs to survive, properly function and avoid getting ill. We need macros in large amounts as they are the primary nutrients for our body. There are three main macronutrients: carbohydrates, proteins, and fats. Micronutrients such as vitamins, minerals, and electrolytes are the other type of nutrients that human body requires, but in comparison to macros, micros are required in much smaller amounts.

Except for fad diets, the human body needs all three macronutrients and cutting out any of the macronutrients puts the risk of nutrient deficiencies and illness on human health.

Carbohydrates that you eat is a source of quick energy, they are transformed into glucose or commonly known as sugar, and are either used right after generated or stored as glycogen for later use.

Protein is there to help with growth, injury repair, muscle formation, and protection against infections. Proteins are the compounds that are built from amino acids, which appear to be the building material for the creation of tissues in the human body. And our body needs 20 various amino acids, 9 of which cannot be produced by our body, and thus must be received from outside sources.

Dietary fat is another essential macronutrient that is responsible for many essential tasks like absorbing the fat-soluble vitamins (A, D, E and K), insulating body during cold weather, surviving long periods without food, protecting organs, supporting cell growth and inducing hormone production.

Usually, to stay healthy, lose weight and for some other reasons we are told to count the number of calories that we intake entirely, forgetting to tell to track macronutrient intake. Calculating and monitoring macronutrient intake can help not only with making health better and reaching fitness goals but can also help you understand which types of foods improve your performance and which are bad for you. If you would like to get such a calculator, you can type in a Google search, and there you will get lots of information on the topic.

Plant-Based Protein Sources

There is a common misconception that vegetarian and vegan diets might be lacking a sufficient amount of protein. However, many dietitians and scientists say that vegetarian or vegan diets have more than enough nutrients in them if planned well. Nevertheless, all foods are different in their protein values, there is food that contains more protein, and there are those that contain less.

Legumes or commonly known as beans have high amounts of protein per serving and contain 15 grams of protein per cooked cup. They are also a great source of iron, complex carbohydrates, folate, fiber, phosphorus, manganese, and potassium. It can be used in a variety of recipes or eaten without anything else.

Nutritional yeast is another excellent source of protein. It has 14 grams of protein per 28 grams. It is also a great source of copper, magnesium, zinc, manganese and all B vitamins. It can be used in a variety of dishes and is sold as flakes and yellow powder.

Next, come lentils. They have 18 grams of protein per cooked cup. They also can be added to a whole variety of dishes. Lentils are also rich in iron, manganese, and folate.

Tempeh, tofu, and edamame are another great source of protein. They are made from whole soybeans, which means they provide all the essential amino acids. All three have 10-19 grams of protein per 100 grams, calcium, and iron. Edamame needs to be steamed or boiled before eating and can be eaten without anything else or incorporated into soups and salads. Tofu and tempeh can also be used in lots of recipes.

Hempseed is another excellent source of protein. It contains 10 grams of protein per 28 grams. It is a good source of iron, magnesium, selenium, zinc, omega-3 and omega-6 fatty acids. It can be added to smoothies, salad dressings, morning muesli, and protein bars.

Spelled and teff are from an ancient grains' category. Teff is gluten-free, whereas spelled contains gluten. They have 10–11 grams of protein per cooked cup. Spelled and teff are rich in iron, zinc, magnesium, selenium, manganese, phosphorus, fiber, B vitamins, and complex carbs. They can be used in a whole variety of dishes.

Spirulina is a blue-green alga and is rich in protein. Two tablespoons will provide 8 grams of protein. It will also cover 22% of the daily iron and thiamin need and 42% of the daily requirement of copper. It is also a good source of riboflavin, magnesium, manganese, essential fatty acids and potassium.

Green peas have 9 grams of protein per cooked cup in them. Green peas are the right choice to get magnesium, iron, zinc, phosphorus, B vitamins and copper. One serving of green peas has enough in it to cover 1/4 of the daily need for vitamin A, C, K, fiber, manganese, folate, and thiamine. It can be used in a whole variety of recipes.

Quinoa and amaranth are ancient or gluten-free grains. They provide 8–9 grams of protein per cooked cup and are complete sources of protein. Amaranth and quinoa are also a good source of iron, complex carbs, fiber, phosphorus, magnesium, and manganese. It can be used in a whole variety of recipes.

Soy milk contains 7 grams of protein per cup and thus a good source of protein, but it's also an excellent source of calcium, vitamin D, and vitamin B12, but only fortified milk contains vitamin B12, so make sure to buy that one. It can be consumed on its own or used in a variety of recipes.

Oats and oatmeal are standard in almost everyone's diet. ½ cup of dry oats provides 6 grams of protein and 4 grams of fiber. It is also a great source of zinc, folate, magnesium, and phosphorus. Oats and oatmeal contain higher-quality protein than rice and wheat. It can be ground into flour and used in a wide variety of recipes as flour and flakes.

Wild rice has more protein than other long-grain rice varieties, including brown rice and basmati. One cooked cup provides 7 grams of protein. It is also a good source of manganese, phosphorus fiber, copper, B vitamins and magnesium. Wild rice is not stripped of its bran and, thus, can contain arsenic in it. Therefore, washing wild rice before cooking is a must, and boiling it in a large amount of water should reduce the possible level of arsenic. It can be used in a wide variety of recipes.

Chia seeds provide 6 grams of protein and 13 grams of fiber per 35 grams. They are also a good source of iron, selenium, calcium, magnesium, antioxidants, and omega-3 fatty acids. It can be used in a wide variety of recipes.

Nuts, seeds, and products from them provide between 5–7 grams of protein per 28 grams. They are also a great source of iron, healthy fats, calcium, fiber, phosphorus, magnesium, vitamin E selenium, specific B vitamins, and antioxidants.

Chapter 12: Protein overview: plant-based proteins, how to calculate them?

It is crucial that we consume a sufficient amount of healthy protein each day to cover our body's requirements. Do you recognize just how much healthy protein you require?

Numerous professional athletes and other people that work out a lot assume that they ought to enhance their healthy protein consumption to assist them to shed their weight or construct even more muscle mass. It is real that the extra you work out, the higher your healthy protein requirement will undoubtedly be.

Healthy protein intake guidelines

Healthy proteins are the standard foundation of the body. They are comprised of amino acids and are required for the formation of muscular tissues, blood, skin, hair, nails, and the wellbeing of the interior body's organs. Besides water, healthy protein is one of the most abundant compounds in the body, and the majority of it is in the skeletal muscle mass.

Considering this, it is assuring to understand that according to the Dietary Guidelines for Americans between 2015-2020, most individuals obtain sufficient healthy protein daily. The very same record directs out that the consumption of fish and shellfish, and plant-based proteins such as seeds and nuts, are frequently lacking.

If you are an athlete, nonetheless, your healthy protein requirements might be somewhat greater considering that resistance training and endurance exercises can swiftly break down muscular tissue healthy protein.

The basic standards for strength-trained and endurance professional athletes, according to the Academy of Nutrition and Dietetics, Dietitians of Canada, and the American College of Sports Medicine, is the recommended amount laying in between 1.2 and 2 grams of healthy protein per kg of body weight to achieve maximum efficiency and the health and wellness of the body.

If you are attempting to gain even more muscular tissue, you might assume that you require a lot healthier protein, yet this isn't what you should do. There is proof that very strict professional athletes or exercisers might take in even more healthy protein (over 3 grams/kilograms daily), but for the typical exerciser, consumption of as much as 2 grams/per kg daily suffices for building muscle mass.

Various ways to determine protein needs

When establishing your healthy protein requirements, you can either recognize a percent of overall day-to-day calories, or you can target in detail the number of grams of healthy protein to eat each day.

Percent of daily calories

Present USDA nutritional standards recommend that adult males and females should take an amount in between 10 and 35 percent of their overall calories intake from healthy protein. To obtain your number and to track your consumption, you'll require to understand the number of calories you eat daily.

To keep a healthy and balanced weight, you need to take in about the same variety of calories that you burn daily.

Just increase that number by 10 percent and by 35 percent to obtain your variety when you understand precisely how many calories you take in daily.

As an example, a male that eats 2,000 calories each day would more or less require to eat between 200 to 700 calories every day of healthy protein.

Healthy protein grams each day

As an option to the portion method, you can target the specific amount of healthy protein grams each day.

One straightforward method to obtain an amount of healthy protein grams daily is to equate the percent array into a particular healthy protein gram variety. The mathematical formula for this is very easy.

Each gram of healthy protein consists of 4 calories, so you will just need to split both calorie array numbers by 4.

A guy that consumes 2,000 calories daily must take in between 200 and 700 calories from healthy protein or 50 to 175 grams of healthy protein.

There are various other methods to obtain a much more specific number which might consider lean muscular tissue mass and/or exercise degree.

You can establish your fundamental healthy protein requirement as a percent of your complete day-to-day calorie consumption or as a series of healthy protein grams daily.

Healthy protein needs based on weight and activity

The ordinary adult demands a minimum of 0.8 grams of healthy protein per kg of body weight each day. One kg equates to 2.2 extra pounds, so an individual that has 165 extra pounds or 75 kg would more or less require around 60 grams of healthy protein daily.

Your healthy protein requirements might raise if you are very active. The Academy of Nutrition and Dietetics, American College of Sports Medicine and the Dietitians of Canada, recommend that professional athletes require even more healthy protein.

They recommend that endurance professional athletes (those that often take part in sports like running, biking, or swimming) take in 1.2 to 1.4 grams of healthy protein per kilo of body weight daily which equates to 0.5 to 0.6 grams of healthy protein per extra pound of body weight.

The companies recommend that strength-trained professional athletes (that engage in exercises like powerlifting or weightlifting often) take in 1.6 to 1.7 grams of healthy protein per kg of body weight. This equates to 0.7 to 0.8 grams of healthy protein per extra pound of body weight.

Healthy protein needs based on lean body mass

A new approach of finding out how much healthy protein you require is focused on the degree of the exercise (how much energy you spend) and your lean body mass. Some professionals really feel that this is an exact extra method because our lean body mass needs extra healthy protein for upkeep than fat.

Lean body mass (LBM) is merely the quantity of bodyweight that is not fat. There are various methods to identify your lean body mass, yet the most convenient is to deduct your body fat from your overall body mass.

You'll require to establish your body fat percent. There are various methods to obtain the number of your body fat consisting of screening with skin calipers, BIA ranges, or DEXA scans. You can approximate your body fat with the following calculating formula.

To determine your overall body fat in extra pounds, you will need to increase your body weight by the body fat portion. If you evaluate yourself to be 150 pounds and that your fat percent is 30, then 45 of those bodyweight pounds would certainly be fat (150 x 30% = 45).

Compute lean body mass. Merely deduct your body fat weight from your overall body weight. Utilizing the exact same instance, the lean body mass would certainly be 105 (150 - 45 = 105).

Calculating your protein needs

While the above standards offer you a general idea of where your healthy protein consumption needs to drop, determining the quantity of day-to-day healthy protein that's right for you, there is another method that can assist you in tweaking the previous results.

To identify your healthy protein requirements in grams (g), you need to initially determine your weight in kgs (kg) by separating your weight in pounds by 2.2.

Next off, choose the number of grams of healthy protein per kilo of bodyweight that is appropriate for you.

Use the reduced end of the array (0.8 g per kg) if you consider yourself to be healthy but not very active.

You should intake a more significant amount of protein (in between 1.2 and 2.0) if you are under tension, expecting, recuperating from a health problem, or if you are associated with extreme and constant weight or endurance training.

(You might require the recommendations of a physician or nutritional expert to assist you to establish this number).

Increase your weight in kg times the number of healthy protein grams per day.

For instance:

A 154-pound man that has as a routine exercising and lifting weights, but is not training at an elite degree:

154 lb/2.2 = 70 kg.

70 kg x 1.7 = 119 grams healthy protein each day.

Healthy protein as a percent of complete calories

An additional means to determine how much healthy protein you require is utilizing your everyday calorie consumption and the percentage of calories that will certainly originate from healthy protein.

Figure out exactly how many calories your body requires each day to keep your current weight.

Discover what your basic metabolic rate (BMR) is by utilizing a BMR calculator (often described as a basic power expense, or BEE, calculator).

Figure out the number of calories you burn via day-to-day tasks and include that number to your BMR.

Next off, choose what portion of your diet plan will certainly originate from healthy protein. The percent you pick will certainly be based upon your objectives, physical fitness degree, age, type of body, and your metabolic rate. The Dietary Guidelines for Americans 2015-2020 advises that healthy protein represent something in between 10 percent and 35 percent for grownups suggested caloric intake.

Multiply that percentage by the complete variety of calories your body requires for the day to establish overall everyday calories from healthy protein.

Split that number by 4. (Quick Reference - 4 calories = 1 gram of healthy protein.)

Chapter 13: Overview of micro and macronutrients

"Will it certainly fit my macros" is a usual statement in the dish preparation and a healthy and balanced way of life room. The attitude is, "I understand specifically what you must be consuming (based upon my customized macronutrient numbers) to shed fat, placed on my muscle mass, or keep weight, after that, it does not matter if you consume pizza, brownies, cookies, or a salad". Is that truly the instance?

You have most likely listened to many talks about macros if you have been in the health and fitness environment for any length of time. Comprehending the truths behind macros and concerning your individual dietary needs will certainly make a difference in your very own wellness journey. In this chapter, we'll discover what macros are, exactly how to recognize if you are consuming the appropriate proportions and the very best foods for supplying them.

Macronutrients are the food classifications that give you the power to bring out our fundamental human features, and they are boiled down right into 3 groups; healthy protein, fats, and carbs. When you recognize precisely how to determine your macros, it is simple to figure out just how much calories you are placing in your body every day and just how much energy you require to burn off the extra calories.

The 3 macronutrients are carbs, fats, and healthy proteins, and they all have various duties in your body. Generally, you'll drop weight. If you desire to obtain an insight into how to monitor your macros, then keep reading.

Carbohydrates:

Composed of starches and sugars, carbohydrates are the macronutrient that your system most calls for. Your body breaks down a lot of carbs as soon as they are ingested, so they are accountable for providing you with an essential source of energy. Unless you get on a specialized consuming strategy like the ketogenic diet plan, carbohydrates ought to compose roughly 45-65% of your caloric requirements.

Not all carbs are developed equivalent, as not all carbs are quickly absorbable or can be used for power manufacturing. Cellulose, as an example, is a non-digestible carb found in vegetables and fruits that serves as a nutritional fiber. This indicates that it aids the body get rid of waste from the big intestinal tract, subsequently maintaining it in functioning order.

Much shorter particles are much easier for your body to break down, so they are identified as basic. Complicated carbohydrates, in comparison, are bigger particles that your body takes longer to break down. In spite of these distinctions, a carbohydrate is a carbohydrate in concerns to your macros.

Healthy protein:

All healthy proteins are made up of mixes of twenty various amino acids, which your body subsequently damages apart and incorporates to develop various physical structures. In other words, your body requires healthy protein to sustain the body's organ performance, power enzyme responses, and to construct your hair, nails, and various other cells.

Of the twenty amino acids, 9 are categorized as necessary, implying that your body cannot produce them, so you require to take them in via food. Those that consume a plant-based diet regimen rather than following an omnivorous diet can likewise satisfy their amino acid requirements by consuming a healthy diet plan that is composed of numerous plant-based resources of healthy protein like nuts, vegetables, and entire grains.

Like carbs, one gram of healthy protein includes 4 calories.

Fat:

In spite of their destructive credibility in previous years, you should not outlaw fats from your diet plan. Your body requires fats to remain healthy and balanced, and in between 10-35% of your food needs to be composed of this macronutrient.

Fats additionally work as a power source, as it is your body's recommended approach for saving extra calories. Your system will just keep percentages of sugar in your cells, yet body fat allows you safe and secure unrestricted amounts of power rather, which you use while resting, throughout the workout, and in between meals.

When you start consuming fats, you are required to guarantee that you provide your system with fats it needs, and that cannot make itself, like omega-3 and omega-6 fats. You can find omega-3s in oily fish, eggs and walnuts, and omega-6s from a lot of veggie oils.

Nutritional fat assists your body to soak up fat-soluble vitamins like A, D, E, and K, and it adds taste and structure to your food. There are 3 main sorts of nutritional fat (hydrogenated fat, unsaturated fat, and trans-fat), and they all have various influences on your wellness.

Hydrogenated fat: found in meat, butter, lotion, and various other animal resources.

It is crucial to keep in mind that you ought to decrease your trans fats intake as much as possible. Frequently called "Franken fats," trans fats can enhance your risks of coronary cardiovascular disease and weight problems.

Water

Water makes up a considerable part of our bodies. It manages our body temperature level and helps in the metabolic process.

The Institute of Medicine suggests drinking 13 cups of water (more or less 3 liters) for males and 9 cups (or 2.2 liters) for females. Not sure if you are getting enough water?

Thinking that calories are the typical means to evaluate your food consumption, why would you take into consideration switching over to grams of macronutrients? The main factor that calories aren't excellent for determining just how healthy and balanced your food options are is that they do not take into consideration what you are consuming. 100 calories of broccoli will certainly rate the exact same as 100 calories of cake, though the 2 could not be more different from a nutritional standpoint.

Changing over to counting your macros, on the other hand, takes top quality food and satiation right into account. By tracking your macro needs, you have a much better possibility of complying with a diet plan that makes good sense for your health and wellness.

How to figure out your macronutrient requirements

While nutritional experts advise particular proportions of each macronutrient for ideal health and wellness, every person's dietary demands will certainly be various. You can identify your specific macronutrient levels with these actions.

1. Identify your calorie requirements:

Your day-to-day calorie requirements depend on lots of variables, including your age, weight, physical fitness level, and a lot more. You can establish your degrees by tracking what you consume in an ordinary week (one in which you aren't shedding or getting weight). The ordinary degree from nowadays is an excellent indication of your calorie requirements.

2. Transform calorie counts to macronutrients

You can designate these calories in the direction of macronutrients based on the proportion you are following when you understand your calorie targets. Frequently, the macronutrient intakes vary between (AMDR) 45-65% of your day-to-day calories from carbohydrates, 20-35% from fats, and 10-35% from healthy protein.

Next off, you can identify the variety of grams to you readily available with standard mathematics. Right here's an instance:

By thinking you require 2,000 calories daily, you can establish your fat consumption by increasing 2,000 by 0.20 (the proportion of fat for 40:40:20 macronutrient divides). That completes 400, which is the variety of daily calories to dedicate to nutritional fat. To establish your gram consumption, divide 400 by 9 (the calories in a gram of fat) for a complete need of 44 grams of fat daily.

Why do individuals count macros?

While we might be used to counting calories, a macro-focused diet plan isn't about the number of calories in your food, instead what sort of calories they are.

"To be healthy and balanced, it is crucial to obtain the best equilibrium of macros in your diet regimen," Dr. Ali states. "Sometimes individuals likewise count macros if they're attempting to drop weight, or for various other factors, such as if they're attempting to ensure they obtain the correct amount of healthy protein they require to get muscular tissue".

Locating that equilibrium suggests recognizing specifically what your body demands and what you intend to acquire or shed. It needs some computations; however, the advantages can be significant.

If It Fits Your Macros (IIFYM) diet regimen merely implies making use of a macro calculator to maintain track of the percent of healthy protein, fats, and the carbohydrates you are consuming.

Is there a fundamental macro calculator anybody can utilize?

Yes ... yet it will undoubtedly need some mathematics.

You require to figure out your basal metabolic rate or BMR. This is the rate at which your body utilizes the energy consumed and differs from one person to another. There are on the internet calculators to aid you with this, or you can do the formula on your own.

For females aged 18-30 it is: 0.0546 x (weight in kilos) + 2.33

For those aged 30-60 it is: 0.0407 x (weight in kilos) + 2.90

You can, after that, use your overall energy expense for a day. If you are much less energetic than the basic population you increase it by 1.49 if you are at an ordinary level, you increase it by 1.63, and if you are much more energetic you increase it by 1.78

That's the number of calories you require each day. Still with me?

From here, you can determine your macro beginning factor. Dr Ali describes: "As a wide estimation, healthy proteins, and carbs, offer us 4 calories for each gram, and fat offers us 9 grams. If you consume a tiny smoked chicken breast, which has 6.4 g of fat and 29g of healthy protein, it would undoubtedly have 58 calories from fat and 116 calories from healthy protein - so 174 calories overall".

"We require around 50% of our calories from carbs, 15% from healthy protein, and 35% from fat, nevertheless, this obviously changes for different people".

"Regardless of whether you are attempting to slim down or construct muscular tissue, you maintain the percentages of 50% carbohydrates, 15% healthy protein, and 35% fat. You would undoubtedly transform the number of calories you would certainly have".

"If you are attempting to slim down, you require 600 calories less than your overall power expense. By doing this, you'll instantly obtain the additional healthy protein and carbohydrate you require to construct muscle mass, yet the percentages continue to be in place".

Applications such as "My Fitness Pal" which has macronutrient rankings and "Fitocracy Macros" are complimentary and can aid you to reach holds with your body's demands and count your macros.

The rationale of the macro diet regimen is that you attempt various dimensions and readjust up until you discover something that matches your needs. The diet plan does not take into account alcohol.

"A glass of rosé can have around 140 calories in it - that's more than a two-finger Ki".

Macronutrient proportions

Now that we've responded to "What are macronutrients?" we need to highlight that like diet plans and health and fitness, macronutrient proportions are not one-size-fits-all. There is no excellent macronutrient proportion that matches every person, and your demands will certainly alter according to various elements in your life.

Each macronutrient has a various calorie degree per gram weight.

Carb = 4 calories per gram.

Healthy protein = 4 calories per gram.

Fat = 9 calories per gram.

The overall calorie net content of food depends on the quantity of carb, healthy protein, and the fat it includes. The thinking was based on the idea that if you get rid of the greater calorie per gram macronutrient, it would certainly be less complicated to minimize the quantity of food.

Chapter 14: Energizing Breakfast

Sweet Potato Toasts

Preparation time: 10 minutes

Cooking time: 10 minutes

Servings: 02

Ingredients:

2 large sweet potatoes, sliced into ¼ inch thick slices

1 tablespoon avocado oil

1 teaspoon salt

½ cup guacamole

½ cup tomatoes, sliced

Directions:

Preheat your oven to 425 degrees F.

Cover a baking sheet with parchment paper.

Rub the potato slices with oil and salt and place them on a baking sheet.

Bake for 5 minutes in the oven, then flip and bake again for 5 minutes.

Top the baked slices with guacamole and tomatoes.

Serve.

Nutrition:

Calories 134

Total Fat 4.7 g

Saturated Fat 0.6 g

Cholesterol 124mg

Sodium 1 mg

Total Carbs 54.1 g

Fiber 7 g

Sugar 3.3 g

Protein 6.2 g

Tofu Scramble Tacos

Preparation time: 10 minutes

Cooking time: 10 minutes

Servings: 04

Ingredients:

1 package tofu

¼ cup nutritional yeast

2 teaspoons garlic powder

2 teaspoons cumin

2 teaspoons chili powder

½ teaspoon turmeric

1 teaspoon salt

½ teaspoon pepper

1 tablespoon avocado oil

Warm corn tortillas

Directions:

In a pan, add avocado oil and tofu.

Sauté and crumble the tofu on medium heat.

Stir in all the remaining spices and yeast.

Mix and cook for 2 minutes.

Serve on tortillas.

Nutrition:

Calories 387

Total Fat 6 g

Saturated Fat 3.4 g

Cholesterol 41 mg

Sodium 154 mg

Total Carbs 37.4 g

Fiber 2.9 g

Sugar 1.3 g

Protein 6.6 g

Almond Chia Pudding

Preparation time: 10 minutes

Cooking time: 0 minutes

Servings: 2

Ingredients:

3 tablespoons almond butter

2 tablespoons maple syrup

1 cup almond milk

¼ cup plus 1 tablespoon chia seeds

Directions:

In a sealable container, add everything and mix well.

Seal the container and refrigerate overnight.

Serve with a splash of almond milk.

Nutrition:

Calories 212

Total Fat 11.8 g

Saturated Fat 2.2 g

Cholesterol 23mg

Sodium 321 mg

Total Carbs 14.6 g

Fibers 4.4 g

Sugar 8 g

Protein 7.3 g

Breakfast Parfait Popsicles

Preparation time: 10 minutes

Cooking time: 0 minutes

Servings: 02

Ingredients:

1 cup soy yogurt

1 cup berries

1 cup granola

Directions:

In a popsicle mold, divide the berries.

Add yogurt to the molds and gently mix the berries using a stick.

Sprinkle granola on top and place the popsicle sticks in the mixture.

Freeze overnight.

Serve.

Nutrition:

Calories 135

Total Fat 2 g

Saturated Fat 1 g

Cholesterol 2 mg

Sodium 17 mg

Total Carbs 33 g

Fiber 1 g

Sugar 13 g

Protein 2 g

Strawberry Smoothie Bowl

Preparation time: 30 minutes

Cooking time: 0 minutes

Servings: 02

Ingredients:

Smoothie bowl:

1½ cups frozen strawberries

½ cup coconut milk

Chia seeds

Directions:

In a blender jug, puree all the ingredients for the smooth bowl.

Pour the smoothie in the serving bowl.

Add strawberries, banana and chia seeds on top.

Chill well then serve.

Nutrition:

Calories 275

Total Fat 14.5 g

Saturated Fat 12.5 g

Cholesterol 36 mg

Sodium 13 mg

Total Carbs 25 g

Fiber 5 g

Sugar 5 g

Protein 2.5 g

Peanut Butter Granola

Preparation time: 10 minutes

Cooking time: 47 minutes

 Servings: 04

Ingredients:

Nonstick spray

4 cups oats

⅓ cup of cocoa powder

¾ cup peanut butter

⅓ cup maple syrup

⅓ cup avocado oil

1½ teaspoons vanilla extract

½ cup cocoa nibs

6 ounces dark chocolate, chopped

Directions:

Preheat your oven to 300 degrees F.

Spray a baking sheet with cooking spray.

In a medium saucepan add oil, maple syrup, and peanut butter.

Cook for 2 minutes on medium heat, stirring.

Add the oats and cocoa powder, mix well.

Spread the coated oats on the baking sheet.

Bake for 45 minutes, occasionally stirring.

Garnish with dark chocolate, cocoa nibs, and peanut butter.

Serve.

Nutrition:

Calories 134

Total Fat 4.7 g

Saturated Fat 0.6 g

Cholesterol 124mg

Sodium 1 mg

Total Carbs 54.1 g

Fiber 7 g

Sugar 3.3 g

Protein 6.2 g

Apple Chia Pudding

Preparation time: 10 minutes

Cooking time: 5 minutes

Servings: 04

Ingredients:

Chia Pudding:

4 tablespoons chia seeds

1 cup almond milk

½ teaspoon cinnamon

Apple Pie Filling:

1 large apple, peeled, cored and chopped

¼ cup water

2 teaspoons maple syrup

Pinch cinnamon

2 tablespoons golden raisins

Directions:

In a sealable container, add cinnamon, chia seeds and almond milk, mix well.

Seal the container and refrigerate overnight.

In a medium pot, combine all apple pie filling ingredients and cook for 5 minutes.

Serve the chia pudding with apple filling on top.

Enjoy.

Nutrition:

Calories 387

Total Fat 5.8 g

Saturated Fat 4.2 g

Cholesterol 41 mg

Sodium 154 mg

Total Carbs 24.1 g

Fiber 2.9 g

Sugar 3.1 g

Protein 6.6 g

Pumpkin Spice Bites

Preparation time: 10 minutes

Cooking time: 0 minutes

Servings: 2

Ingredients:

½ cup pumpkin puree

½ cup almond butter

¼ cup maple syrup

1 teaspoon pumpkin pie spice

1⅓ cup rolled oats

⅓ cup pumpkin seeds

⅓ cup raisins

2 tablespoons chia seeds

Directions:

In a sealable container, add everything and mix well.

Seal the container and refrigerate overnight.

Roll the mixture into small balls.

Serve.

Nutrition:

Calories 212

Total Fat 11.8 g

Saturated Fat 2.2 g

Cholesterol 23mg

Sodium 321 mg

Total Carbs 14.6 g

Fibers 4.4 g

Sugar 8 g

Protein 7.3 g

Lemon Spelt Scones

Preparation time: 10 minutes

Cooking time: 18 minutes

Servings: 6

Ingredients:

1¾ cups spelt flour

1¼ cup whole spelt

⅔ cup coconut sugar

2 teaspoons baking powder

½ teaspoon salt

3 tablespoons lemon zest

½ cup coconut oil

1 cup coconut cream

2 tablespoons almond milk

2 cups frozen raspberries

Directions:

Preheat your oven to 425 degrees F.

Whisk dry ingredients in a stand mixer using whisk attachment.

Freeze the dry mixture for 10 minutes then place it back on the mixer.

Using the paddle attachment, stir in coconut oil, coconut cream, and almond milk then beat until smooth.

Fold in frozen raspberries and mix again, divide the dough into two parts. Spread each part into a thick disk and cut each into 6 wedges of equal size. Line a suitable baking sheet with parchment paper and place the wedges on the tray.

Bake for 18 minutes then serve.

Nutrition:

Calories 119

Total Fat 14 g

Saturated Fat 2 g

Cholesterol 65 mg

Sodium 269 mg

Total Carbs 19 g

Fiber 4 g

Sugar 6 g

Protein 5g

Veggie Breakfast Scramble

Preparation time: 10 minutes

Cooking time: 14 minutes

Servings: 06

Ingredients:

1 cup yellow onions, chopped

1 cup red bell peppers, diced

1½ cups zucchini, sliced

3 cups cauliflower florets

1 tablespoon garlic, minced

1 tablespoon tamari

2 tablespoons vegetable broth

2 tablespoons nutritional yeast

1 (15 ounce) can chickpeas, drained

2 cups baby spinach, chopped

Spice Mix:

1 teaspoon onion powder

1 teaspoon garlic powder

1 teaspoon dried minced onions

¾ teaspoon dried ground mustard powder

1 teaspoon dried thyme leaves

1 teaspoon smoked paprika

¼ teaspoon turmeric

¾ teaspoon salt

¼ teaspoon black pepper

Directions:

In a suitable pan, add cooking oil and all the vegetables.

Cook while stirring for 7 minutes on medium heat.

Toss in the chickpeas and all the spices.

Continue sautéing for another 7 minutes.

Serve warm.

Nutrition:

Calories 231

Total Fat 20.1 g

Saturated Fat 2.4 g

Cholesterol 110 mg

Sodium 941 mg

Total Carbs 20.1 g

Fiber 0.9 g

Sugar 1.4 g

Protein 4.6 g

Chapter 15: Sauces, soups and grains

Wine Sauce

Preparation Time: 15 minutes

Cooking Time: 10 minutes

 Servings: 8

Ingredients:

1 tablespoon olive oil

1 shallot, minced

3 tablespoons freshly squeezed lemon juice

¼ cup dry white wine

½ teaspoon lemon zest

1 tablespoon parsley, chopped

1 tablespoon capers, chopped

1 cup chicken broth

Salt and pepper to taste

1 tablespoon cornstarch

2 tablespoons butter

Directions:

Pour the oil into a pan over medium heat.

Cook the shallot for 1 minute.

Pour in the lemon juice and wine.

Stir in the zest.

Bring to a boil.

Simmer for 3 to 5 minutes.

Add the parsley, capers and broth.

Season with salt and pepper.

Cook for 5 minutes.

Mix the cornstarch and water.

Stir the cornstarch mixture into the sauce.

Add the butter and cook until melted.

Refrigerate for up to 3 days.

Nutritional Value:

Calories: 46

Total fat: 3.2g

Saturated fat: 1.1g

Cholesterol: 4mg

Sodium: 116mg

Potassium: 51mg

Carbohydrates: 2.8g

Fiber: 0.1g

Sugar: 1g

Protein: 0.6g

Garlic and White Bean Soup

Cooking time: 10 minutes

Servings: 4

Ingredients:

45 ounces cooked cannellini beans

1/4 teaspoon dried thyme

2 teaspoons minced garlic

1/8 teaspoon crushed red pepper

1/2 teaspoon dried rosemary

1/8 teaspoon ground black pepper

2 tablespoons olive oil

4 cups vegetable broth

Directions:

Place one-third of white beans in a food processor, then pour in 2 cups broth and pulse for 2 minutes until smooth.

Place a pot over medium heat, add oil and when hot, add garlic and cook for 1 minute until fragrant.

Add pureed beans into the pan along with remaining beans, sprinkle with spices and herbs, pour in the broth, stir until combined, and bring the mixture to boil over medium-high heat.

Switch heat to medium-low level, simmer the beans for 15 minutes, and then mash them with a fork.

Taste the soup to adjust seasoning and then serve.

Nutrition:

Calories: 222 Cal

Fat: 7 g

Carbs: 13 g

Protein: 11.2 g

Fiber: 9.1 g

Coconut Curry Lentils

Preparation time: 10 minutes

Cooking time: 40 minutes

Servings: 4

Ingredients:

1 cup brown lentils

1 small white onion, peeled, chopped

1 teaspoon minced garlic

1 teaspoon grated ginger

3 cups baby spinach

1 tablespoon curry powder

2 tablespoons olive oil

13 ounces coconut milk, unsweetened

2 cups vegetable broth

For Serving:

4 cups cooked rice

1/4 cup chopped cilantro

Directions:

Place a large pot over medium heat, add oil and when hot, add ginger and garlic and cook for 1 minute until fragrant.

Add onion, cook for 5 minutes, stir in curry powder, cook for 1 minute until toasted, add lentils and pour in broth.

Switch heat to medium-high level, bring the mixture to a boil, then switch heat to the low level and simmer for 20 minutes until tender and all the liquid is absorbed.

Pour in milk, stir until combined, turn heat to medium level, and simmer for 10 minutes until thickened.

Then remove the pot from heat, stir in spinach, let it stand for 5 minutes until its leaves wilts and then top with cilantro.

Serve lentils with rice.

Nutrition:

Calories: 184 Cal

Fat: 3.7 g

Carbs: 30 g

Protein: 11.3 g

Fiber: 10.7 g

Tuscan Tomato and Bread Soup

Preparation time 5 minutes

cook time: 50 minutes

Servings: 4 servings

Ingredients:

4 cups cubed Italian bread

1/4 cup olive oil

4 garlic cloves, minced

1 (28-ounce) can crushed tomatoes

2 fresh ripe tomatoes, cut into 1/2-inch dice

4 cups vegetable broth or water

2 tablespoons minced fresh parsley

Salt and freshly ground black pepper

Torn fresh basil leaves, for garnish

Directions:

In a large soup pot over medium heat, heat 2 tablespoons of the oil. Add the garlic and cook until softened, about 1 minute. Stir in the canned and fresh tomatoes, broth, parsley, and salt and pepper to taste. Bring to a boil, then reduce heat to low and simmer for 30 minutes.

Divide the toasted bread among 4 bowls and ladle the soup over the bread. The bread should absorb most of the liquid in the soup. Garnish with basil leaves, drizzle with the remaining 2 tablespoons oil, and serve.

Nutrition:

Calories 134

Total Fat 4.7 g

Saturated Fat 0.6 g

Cholesterol 124mg

Sodium 1 mg

Total Carbs 54.1 g

Fiber 7 g

Sugar 3.3 g

Protein 6.2 g

Moroccan vermicelli vegetable soup

Preparation time 5 minutes

cook time: 35 minutes

Servings: 4 to 6 servings

Ingredients

1 tablespoon olive oil

1 small onion, chopped

1 large carrot, chopped

1 celery rib, chopped

3 small zucchinis, cut into 1/4-inch dice

1 (28-ounce) can diced tomatoes, drained

2 tablespoons tomato paste

1½ cups cooked or 1 (15.5-ounce) can chickpeas, drained and rinsed

2 teaspoons smoked paprika

1 teaspoon ground cumin

1 teaspoon za'atar spice (optional)

1/4 teaspoon ground cayenne

6 cups vegetable broth, homemade (see light vegetable broth) or store-bought, or water

Salt

4 ounces vermicelli

2 tablespoons minced fresh cilantro, for garnish

Directions

In a large soup pot, heat the oil over medium heat. Add the onion, carrot, and celery. Cover and cook until softened, about 5 minutes. Stir in the zucchini, tomatoes, tomato paste, chickpeas, paprika, cumin, za'atar, and cayenne. Add the broth and salt to taste. Bring to a boil, then reduce heat to low and simmer, uncovered, until the vegetables are tender, about 30 minutes.

Shortly before serving, stir in the vermicelli and cook until the noodles are tender, about 5 minutes. Ladle the soup into bowls, garnish with cilantro, and serve.

Nutrition:

Calories 134

Total Fat 4.7 g

Saturated Fat 0.6 g

Cholesterol 124mg

Sodium 1 mg

Total Carbs 54.1 g

Fiber 7 g

Sugar 3.3 g

Protein 6.2 g

Black bean and corn salad with cilantro dressing

Preparation time 15 minutes

cook time: 0 minutes

 Servings: 4 servings

Ingredients:

2 cups frozen corn, thawed

3 cups cooked or 2 (15.5-ounce) cans black beans, rinsed and drained

1/2 cup chopped red bell pepper

1/4 cup minced red onion

1 (4-ounce) can chopped mild green chiles, drained

2 garlic cloves, crushed

1/4 cup chopped fresh cilantro

1 teaspoon ground cumin

1/2 teaspoon salt (optional)

1/4 teaspoon freshly ground black pepper

2 tablespoons fresh lime juice

2 tablespoons water

1/4 cup olive oil

Directions:

In a blender or food processor, mince the garlic. Add the cilantro, cumin, salt, and black pepper and pulse to blend. Add the lime juice, water, and oil and process until well blended. Pour the dressing over the salad and toss to combine. Taste, adjusting seasonings if necessary, and serve.

Nutrition:

Calories 134

Total Fat 7 g

Saturated Fat 0.6 g

Cholesterol 14mg

Sodium 1 mg

Total Carb 4.1 g

Fiber 7 g

Sugar 3 g

Protein 6.2 g

Black beans and wild rice

Preparation time 5 minutes

cook time: 50 minutes

Servings: 4 servings

Ingredients:

¾ cup wild rice

1 teaspoon dried marjoram

½ teaspoon salt

¼ teaspoon freshly ground black pepper

3 cups fresh baby spinach

Directions:

Combine the wild rice in a large saucepan with 3 cups of salted water. Bring to a boil, then reduce heat to low, cover, and simmer for 40 minutes or until tender. Add the beans, tomatoes, marjoram, salt, and pepper.

Cover and cook over low heat, stirring occasionally, until the flavors are well combined, about 15 minutes, adding a splash of water if too dry.

Stir in the spinach and cook until the spinach is wilted and the flavors have blended, about 5 minutes. Taste, adjusting seasonings if necessary. Serve immediately.

Nutrition:

Calories 164

Total Fat 4.7 g

Saturated Fat 0.6 g

Cholesterol 124mg

Sodium 1 mg

Total Carbs 54.1 g

Fiber 7 g

Sugar 3.3 g

Protein 6.2 g

Orange & honey sauce

Preparation time: 15 minutes

cooking time: 15 minutes

servings: 8

Ingredients:

1 tablespoon olive oil

¼ cup chopped shallot

¼ cup freshly squeezed orange juice

½ teaspoon orange zest

1 cup champagne

1 tablespoon honey

Salt and pepper to taste

¼ teaspoon ground coriander

1 tablespoon cornstarch

2 tablespoons dry white wine

1 tablespoon butter

Directions:

Pour the oil into a pan over medium heat.

Cook the shallot for 1 minute.

Stir in the orange juice, orange zest, champagne, honey, salt, pepper and coriander.

Bring to a boil. Cook for 10 minutes.

In a bowl, mix the cornstarch and wine.

Add this mixture to the pan.

Stir in butter and cook until melted.

Refrigerate for up to 3 days.

Nutritional value:

Calories: 83

Total fat: 3.2g

Saturated fat: 1.1g

Cholesterol: 4mg

Sodium: 74mg

Potassium: 35mg

Carbohydrates: 5.5g

Fiber: 0.1g

Sugar: 3g

Protein: 0.4g

Butternut squash sauce

Preparation time: 10 minutes

cooking time: 13 minutes

 servings: 12

Ingredients:

2 cups water

½ cup cashew, chopped

2 tablespoons olive oil

2 sweet onions, diced

2 tablespoons garlic, minced

½ teaspoon salt

¼ cup dry white wine

¾ teaspoon dried oregano

1 cup butternut squash puree

⅛ teaspoon ground nutmeg

Pepper to taste

Directions:

Blend cashews and water in a food processor until smooth. Set aside.

Pour the oil into a pan over medium heat.

Cook the onion and garlic for 3 minutes.

Season with salt.

Reduce heat and cook for another 10 minutes.

Stir in the wine and oregano.

Add the squash puree, nutmeg and cashew.

Cook for 3 minutes.

Refrigerate for up to 3 days.

Nutritional Value:

Calories: 102

Total fat: 5.3g

Saturated fat: 0.9g

Sodium: 184mg

Potassium: 216mg

Carbohydrates: 10.9g

Fiber: 2.1g

Sugar: 4g

Protein: 1.8g

Comfort Soup

Servings: 5-6

Preparation Time: 5 minutes

Cooking Time: 35 minutes

Ingredients:

½ cups of freshly diced onion 1 teaspoon of paprika

½ tablespoon of water

3 ½ cups of water

1 cup of freshly diced carrots 3 freshly minced large cloves of garlic 1 cup of freshly diced celery 1 teaspoon of mild curry powder 2 cups of dried red lentils

½ teaspoon of sea salt

Freshly ground black pepper to taste ¼ teaspoon of dried thyme

3 cups of vegetable stock

1 – 1 ½ teaspoons of lemon juice/apple cider vinegar 2 teaspoons of freshly chopped rosemary

Directions:

Put a large pot on the stove over medium heat.

Add 1 ½ teaspoons of water along with celery, onion, carrot, paprika, garlic, curry powder, sea salt, black pepper, and thyme.

After all the herbs and spices are inside the pot, cover them and cook for about 7-8 minutes, stirring occasionally so that the spices do not burn.

Rinse the lentils and add them to 3 ½ cups of water. Stir into the stock.

Cover the pot and allow everything to simmer for 12-15 minutes.

Add the rosemary and simmer for another 10 minutes. You will know that your soup is ready when the lentils are fully softened.

Add the vinegar and some more water, if you want a thinner liquid.

Serve the soup with your favorite bread.

If you do not have fresh rosemary, you can also add dried rosemary. In that case, add it with the rest of the herbs and spices at the beginning. You can use ½ to 1 teaspoon of dried rosemary.

Nutrition:

Fat – 5 g

Protein – 7.6 g

Carbohydrate – 23 g

Chapter 16: High protein Salads

Antioxidant Kale Salad

Servings Four

Preparation time Ten Minutes

Ingredients:

Kale 3 C.

Dried Cranberries .50 C.

Fresh Raspberries 2 C.

Blueberries 2 C.

Carrots 1, Shredded

Almonds .25 C.

Directions:

This salad is lovely to add to any diet because it is full of flavor and offers a boost of nutrition. Before you assemble your salad, make sure you wash the fruit and vegetables.

When you are all set, toss together the ingredients in a mixing bowl, top with your dressing, and your salad is ready to be served.

Nutritional value:

Calories: 83

Total fat: 3.2g

Saturated fat: 1.1g

Cholesterol: 4mg

Sodium: 74mg

Potassium: 35mg

Carbohydrates: 5.5g

Fiber: 0.1g

Sugar: 3g

Protein: 0.4g

Beet and Kale Salad

Servings: 2

Preparation Time: 5 minutes

Cooking Time: 5 minutes

Ingredients:

8 ounces of beet and kale blend 1 tablespoon of olive oil

1 cucumber

13.4 ounce of chickpeas

Salt

2 tablespoons of red wine vinegar Pepper

¼ cup of walnuts

2 ounces of dried cranberries Cashew cheese

Directions

Cut the veggies and combine everything in a big salad bowl.

Nutrition:

Fat – 24 g

Carbohydrates – 65 g

Protein – 24 g

Kale and Cauliflower Salad

Servings: 2

Calories: 430 per serving Preparation Time: 10 minutes Cooking Time: 15 minutes

Ingredients:

6 ounces of Lacinato kale

8 ounces of cauliflower florets 1 lemon

1 tablespoon of Italian spice 2 radishes

13.4 ounce of butter beans

Olive oil

¼ cup of walnuts

¼ cup of vegan Caesar dressing Pepper

Salt

Nutrition:

Fat – 15 g

Carbohydrates – 41 g

Protein – 18 g

Directions:

Preheat the oven to 400°F. Put the cauliflower florets on a baking sheet, toss them with olive oil and spices, and add salt. Roast the cauliflower until it is brown. It will be done within 15-20 minutes.

De-stem the kale and slice the leaves. Slice the radishes. Both kale and radish should be sliced thinly. Cut the lemon in half.

Put the kale in a large bowl and add the lemon juice and salt along with the pepper. Massage the kale so that it is properly covered with seasoning. The leaves will soon turn dark green. Mix the radishes.

Rinse the butter beans and pat them dry with a towel. On medium-high heat, put a large skillet, add some olive oil, and sauté the butter beans in a layer. Sprinkle some salt on top and shake the pan. The butter beans will be brown in places within 7 minutes.

Take two large plates and divide both the kale and beans equally. Put the walnuts and roasted cauliflower on top. Add the Caesar dressing on top and enjoy the amazing salad.

Nutritional value:

Calories: 83

Total fat: 3.2g

Saturated fat: 1.1g

Cholesterol: 4mg

Sodium: 74mg

Potassium: 35mg

Carbohydrates: 5.5g

Fiber: 0.1g

Sugar: 3g

Protein: 0.4g

Asian Delight with Crunchy Dressing

Servings: 4

Preparation Time: 20 minutes

Cooking Time: 10 minutes

Ingredients:

Salad Dressing

½ teaspoon of powdered ginger or 1 teaspoon of freshly chopped ginger 1 tablespoon of honey

¼ cup of rice wine vinegar

2 tablespoons of soy sauce

3 tablespoons of sesame oil

3 tablespoons of creamy peanut butter ¼ cup of vegetable oil

2 tablespoons of toasted sesame seeds Salad

1 finely shredded carrot

1 thinly sliced red bell pepper 6 cups of washed and dried spinach ¼ thinly sliced red onion

1 thinly sliced cucumber

½ pound of snap peas

½ cup of roasted peanuts

1 tablespoon of toasted sesame seeds

Directions:

In a medium bowl, mix the dressing ingredients and whisk them well. Do not put the sesame seeds in this dressing mixture.

Put some water in the pot and bring it to a boil. Add the sugar snap peas and cook them for about 5 minutes until they are crisp and tender. Drain and rinse them repeatedly in cold water so that the peas retain their crispy nature.

In a large bowl, add all the other ingredients for the salad. Put the salad dressing on top so that the veggies are well-coated. Add the toasted sesame seeds. Enjoy this salad when you are not in the mood for anything heavy.

Nutrition:

Fat – 42 g

Carbohydrates – 23 g

Protein – 13 g

Broccoli Salad the Thai Way

Servings: 2

Preparation Time: 10 minutes

Cooking Time: 25 minutes

Ingredients:

1 tablespoon of tamari

¾ cup of mung beans

1 lime

2 garlic cloves

3 tablespoons of cashew butter 1 cucumber

¼ ounce of fresh mint

1 tablespoon of chili-garlic sauce 1 head of artisan lettuce

3 Thai chilis

6 ounces of broccoli florets

2 tablespoons of olive oil

Salt

Pepper

Directions:

On high heat, add the mung beans to 3 cups of cold water. After they start boiling, reduce the heat to medium. Allow the beans to simmer, but stir them from time to time. The mung beans will be tender within 20 minutes. Drain the excess water and add some salt.

Mince the garlic and cut the lime in half. In a medium bowl, mix the lime juice, minced garlic, tamari, and cashew butter with chili-garlic sauce. Add 3 tablespoons of warm water. Whisk the mixture well.

Slice the cucumber, cut the broccoli into bite-size pieces, and chop the lettuce. Pick the mint leaves as well. Lastly, slice the Thai chilis.

On a non-stick skillet, put 2 tablespoons of olive oil. Turn the heat to medium-high. Once the oil is hot, add the broccoli florets and cook until they are brown. They will be crisp-tender. Add some pepper and salt to the broccoli and add the lime juice and Thai chilis.

In a shallow bowl, spread some cashew sauce. Add some chopped lettuce, mung beans, broccoli, and cucumber. Add mint leaves and mix the Thai chilies. Add some more cashew sauce and enjoy the salad!

Nutrition:

Fat – 13 g

Carbohydrates – 62 g

Protein – 25 g

Citrus Tomato Salad

Servings Four

Preparation time Ten Minutes

Ingredients:

Mixed Greens 3 C.

Avocado 1, Diced

Tomatoes 2 C., Diced

Lime Juice 1 T.

Onion .50 C., Diced

Parsley 1 T.

Directions:

Tomato and lime juice go together surprisingly well! If you are looking for a slightly different salad, give this one a chance!

Begin by chopping up the avocado, tomatoes, and onion the way directed and place on top of your mixed greens. Once you have tossed everything together well, you will want to sprinkle the parsley over the top, drip some lime juice in, and then enjoy your salad.

Nutrition:

Fat – 13 g

Carbohydrates – 62 g

Protein – 25 g

Classic Kale Salad

Servings Three

Preparation time Ten Minutes

Ingredients:

Kale 3 C.

Pine Nuts .10 C.

Walnuts .10 C.

Quinoa 1 C.

Olives 1 C.

Directions:

The first step in recreating this salad will be cooking the quinoa. You will want to complete this by following the guidelines that are provided on the package. Generally, this should only take you ten to fifteen minutes. When the quinoa is cooked to your liking, place it into a salad bowl with the rest of the ingredients.

As a final touch, you will want to find a plant-based Caesar dressing or any of your favorites. After you have given the salad a good toss, it will be all set to be served for your next meal.

Nutrition:

Fat – 32 g

Carbohydrates – 42 g

Protein – 5 g

Creamy Tahini Chickpea Salad

Servings Four

Preparation time Ten Minutes

Ingredients:

Tahini Paste 2 T.

Chickpeas 1 Can

Lemon Juice 2 T.

Shallot 1, Minced

Pepper Dash

Directions:

This recipe offers an alternative to potato salad or tuna salad. If you like something creamy for your sandwiches or as a side, this recipe is perfect for you.

To recreate this salad, you will place your chickpeas into a bowl and gently combine the lemon juice and tahini paste in until the chickpeas are well coated.

Once the chickpeas are coated, add in the shallot pieces and dash with pepper to your liking. When the dish is seasoned to your liking, it can be served.

Nutrition:

Fat – 13 g

Carbohydrates – 62 g

Protein – 25 g

Chilled Winter Salad

Servings Five

Preparation time Ten Minutes

Ingredients:

Arugula 3 C.

Parsley 2 C.

Spinach 3 C.

Garlic Cloves 1, Minced

Onion .50, Sliced

Cabbage .50, Shredded

Red Wine Vinegar .33 C.

Directions:

Don't let the title fool you; this salad can be enjoyed during any season of the year! It is called a winter salad simply because of the available ingredients.

When you want to make this salad, you can place all of the ingredients into your serving bowl and toss together. Once this step is complete, add in some red wine vinegar, and it will be ready for your enjoyment.

Nutrition:

Fat – 10 g

Carbohydrates – 12 g

Protein – 5 g

Simple Superfood Salad

Servings Two

Preparation time Five Minutes

Ingredients:

Kale 3 C.

Tomatoes .50 C.

Carrots 1, Sliced

Blueberries .25 C.

Vinaigrette Salad Dressing 3 T.

Directions:

If you need to whip a salad together as quickly as possible, this is going to be the perfect recipe for you to do so. Before you assemble the salad, be sure to slice and dice your tomatoes and carrots beforehand. Once this step is complete, add everything into a bowl and coat with the salad dressing before serving up.

Nutrition:

Fat – 3 g

Carbohydrates – 2 g

Protein – 5 g

Krunchy Kale Salad

Servings Four

Preparation time Ten Minutes

Ingredients:

Kale 3 C.

Lemon Juice 3 T.

Walnuts .25 C., Chopped

Pear 1, Chopped

Pepper Dash

Directions:

It isn't every day that you see fresh pear in a salad! Between the crunch of the walnuts and the citrus flavor of the lemon juice, this salad is very refreshing.

All you are going to have to do add all of the items into your bowl, season to your liking, and then it will be set for your enjoyment.

Nutrition:

Fat – 17 g

Carbohydrates – 72 g

Protein – 25 g

Chapter 17: Smoothies and Drinks

Mango strawberry smoothie

Preparation time: 5 minutes

Cooking time: 5 minutes

Servings: 2

Ingredients:

1 cup strawberry sliced

6-ounce plain yogurt

A mango sliced

6-8 ice cubes

Directions:

Take a blender. Add mango cubes, strawberries, ice and yogurt. Blend all ingredients well until smooth and even. Pour more ice if required and blend again until a fine texture is obtained. Pour into serving glasses. Serve chilled and refreshing smoothie. Nutrition:

Fat – 10 g

Carbohydrates – 2 g

Protein – 25 g

Honeydew kiwi cooler

Preparation time: 5 minutes

Cooking time: 5 minutes

Servings: 2

Ingredients:

2 cup honeydew melon

1 tbsp. lemon juice

1 tbsp. honey

3 ice cubes

½ cup frozen kiwi

Directions:

In a blender, add honeydew, lemon juice, honey and blend until smooth. After that, add ice cubes and blend again until the desired consistency is obtained. Now add kiwi and give a pulse that the kiwi is broken but don't blend its seeds. Pour the smoothie in serving glasses and serve chilled.

Nutrition:

Fat – 17 g

Carbohydrates – 72 g

Protein – 25 g

Frosty cappuccino

Preparation time: 5 minutes

Cooking time: 5 minutes

Servings:2

Ingredients:

1 cup low-fat milk

1 tsp espresso coffee powder

1 tbsp. Chocolate syrup

2 ice cubes

Sugar as per taste

1 tsp cinnamon

Directions: Take a blender. Pour milk, chocolate syrup, espresso powder and blend until well combined. Now add ice cubes and blend to make smooth and frothy. Add sugar to taste and pulse for a few seconds. Pour into serving glasses and garnish with cinnamon powder. Serve the chill frosty cappuccino. Nutrition:

Fat – 17 g

Carbohydrates – 2 g

Protein – 5 g

Apricot-raspberry refresher

Preparation time: 5 minutes

Cooking time: 5 minutes

Servings: 2

Ingredients:

1cup apricot nectar

1 tbsp. honey

½ cup apricot halved

¼ cup frozen raspberries

3 ice cubes

Directions:

Take a blender. Add apricot, apricot nectar, honey and blend to make a smooth consistency. Now add ice cubes and blend again. At last, add raspberries and pulse for a few seconds but not to make a smooth consistency. Pour into smoothie glasses and serve chilled.

Nutrition:

Fat – 17 g

Carbohydrates – 72 g

Protein – 25 g

Mexican Hot Chocolate Mix

Preparation time: 5 minutes

Cooking time: 0 minute

Servings: 2

Ingredients: For the Hot Chocolate Mix:

1/3 cup chopped dark chocolate

1/8 teaspoon cayenne

1/8 teaspoon salt

1/2 teaspoon cinnamon

1/4 cup coconut sugar

1 teaspoon cornstarch

3 tablespoons cocoa powder

1/2 teaspoon vanilla extract, unsweetened

For Serving:

2 cups milk, warmed

Directions:

Place all the ingredients of hot chocolate mix in the order in a food processor or blender and then pulse for 2 to 3 minutes at high speed until ground.

Stir 2 tablespoons of the chocolate mix into a glass of milk until combined and then serve.

Nutrition:

Calories: 127 Cal

Fat: 5 g

Carbs: 20 g

Protein: 1 g

Fiber: 2 g

Pumpkin Spice Frappuccino

Preparation time: 5 minutes

Cooking time: 0 minute

Servings: 2

Ingredients:

½ teaspoon ground ginger

1/8 teaspoon allspice

½ teaspoon ground cinnamon

2 tablespoons coconut sugar

1/8 teaspoon nutmeg

¼ teaspoon ground cloves

1 teaspoon vanilla extract, unsweetened

2 teaspoons instant coffee

2 cups almond milk, unsweetened

1 cup of ice cubes

Directions:

Place all the ingredients in the order in a food processor or blender and then pulse for 2 to 3 minutes at high speed until smooth.

Pour the Frappuccino into two glasses and then serve.

Nutrition:

Calories: 90 Cal

Fat: 6 g

Carbs: 5 g

Protein: 2 g

Fiber: 1 g

Cookie Dough Milkshake

Preparation time: 5 minutes

Cooking time: 0 minute

Servings: 2

Ingredients:

2 tablespoons cookie dough

5 dates, pitted

2 teaspoons chocolate chips

1/2 teaspoon vanilla extract, unsweetened

1/2 cup almond milk, unsweetened

1 ½ cup almond milk ice cubes

Directions:

Place all the ingredients in the order in a food processor or blender and then pulse for 2 to 3 minutes at high speed until smooth.

Pour the milkshake into two glasses and then serve with some cookie dough balls.

Nutrition:

Calories: 208 Cal

Fat: 9 g

Carbs: 30 g

Protein: 2 g

Fiber: 2 g

Strawberry and Hemp Smoothie

Preparation time: 5 minutes

Cooking time: 0 minute

Servings: 2

Ingredients:

3 cups fresh strawberries

2 tablespoons hemp seeds

1/2 teaspoon vanilla extract, unsweetened

1/8 teaspoon sea salt

2 tablespoons maple syrup

1 cup vegan yogurt

1 cup almond milk, unsweetened

1 cup of ice cubes

2 tablespoons hemp protein

Directions:

Place all the ingredients in the order in a food processor or blender, except for protein powder, and then pulse for 2 to 3 minutes at high speed until smooth.

Pour the smoothie into two glasses and then serve.

Nutrition:

Calories: 258 Cal

Fat: 17 g

Carbs: 12 g

Protein: 14 g

Fiber: 2 g

Blueberry, Hazelnut and Hemp Smoothie

Preparation time: 5 minutes

Cooking time: 0 minute

Servings: 2

Ingredients:

2 tablespoons hemp seeds

1 ½ cups frozen blueberries

2 tablespoons chocolate protein powder

1/2 teaspoon vanilla extract, unsweetened

2 tablespoons chocolate hazelnut butter

1 small frozen banana

3/4 cup almond milk

Directions:

Place all the ingredients in the order in a food processor or blender and then pulse for 2 to 3 minutes at high speed until smooth.

Pour the smoothie into two glasses and then serve.

Nutrition:

Calories: 376 Cal

Fat: 25 g

Carbs: 26 g

Protein: 14 g

Fiber: 4 g

Mango Lassi

Preparation time: 5 minutes

Cooking time: 0 minute

Servings: 2

Ingredients:

1 ¼ cup mango pulp

1 tablespoon coconut sugar

1/8 teaspoon salt

1/2 teaspoon lemon juice

1/4 cup almond milk, unsweetened

1/4 cup chilled water

1 cup cashew yogurt

Directions:

Place all the ingredients in the order in a food processor or blender and then pulse for 2 to 3 minutes at high speed until smooth.

Pour the lassi into two glasses and then serve.

Nutrition:

Calories: 218 Cal

Fat: 2 g

Carbs: 44 g

Protein: 3 g

Fiber: 1 g

Mocha Chocolate Shake

Preparation time: 5 minutes

Cooking time: 0 minute

Servings: 2

Ingredients:

1/4 cup hemp seeds

2 teaspoons cocoa powder, unsweetened

1/2 cup dates, pitted

1 tablespoon instant coffee powder

2 tablespoons flax seeds

2 1/2 cups almond milk, unsweetened

1/2 cup crushed ice

Directions:

Place all the ingredients in the order in a food processor or blender and then pulse for 2 to 3 minutes at high speed until smooth.

Pour the smoothie into two glasses and then serve.

Nutrition:

Calories: 357 Cal

Fat: 21 g

Carbs: 31 g

Protein: 12 g

Fiber: 5 g

Chard, Lettuce and Ginger Smoothie

Preparation time: 5 minutes

Cooking time: 0 minute

Servings: 2

Ingredients:

10 Chard leaves, chopped

1-inch piece of ginger, chopped

10 lettuce leaves, chopped

½ teaspoon black salt

2 pears, chopped

2 teaspoons coconut sugar

¼ teaspoon ground black pepper

¼ teaspoon salt

2 tablespoons lemon juice

2 cups of water

Directions:

Place all the ingredients in the order in a food processor or blender and then pulse for 2 to 3 minutes at high speed until smooth.

Pour the smoothie into two glasses and then serve.

Nutrition:

Calories: 514 Cal

Fat: 0 g

Carbs: 15 g

Protein: 4 g

Fiber: 4 g

Red Beet, Pear and Apple Smoothie

Preparation time: 5 minutes

Cooking time: 0 minute

Servings: 2

Ingredients:

1/2 of medium beet, peeled, chopped

1 tablespoon chopped cilantro

1 orange, juiced

1 medium pear, chopped

1 medium apple, cored, chopped

1/4 teaspoon ground black pepper

1/8 teaspoon rock salt

1 teaspoon coconut sugar

1/4 teaspoons salt

1 cup of water

Directions:

Place all the ingredients in the order in a food processor or blender and then pulse for 2 to 3 minutes at high speed until smooth.

Pour the smoothie into two glasses and then serve.

Nutrition:

Calories: 132 Cal

Fat: 0 g

Carbs: 34 g

Protein: 1 g

Fiber: 5 g

Berry and Yogurt Smoothie

Preparation time: 5 minutes

Cooking time: 0 minute

Servings: 2

Ingredients:

2 small bananas

3 cups frozen mixed berries

1 ½ cup cashew yogurt

1/2 teaspoon vanilla extract, unsweetened

1/2 cup almond milk, unsweetened

Directions:

Place all the ingredients in the order in a food processor or blender and then pulse for 2 to 3 minutes at high speed until smooth.

Pour the smoothie into two glasses and then serve.

Nutrition:

Calories: 326 Cal

Fat: 6.5 g

Carbs: 65.6 g

Protein: 8 g

Fiber: 8.4 g

Chocolate and Cherry Smoothie

Preparation time: 5 minutes

Cooking time: 0 minute

Servings: 2

Ingredients:

4 cups frozen cherries

2 tablespoons cocoa powder

1 scoop of protein powder

1 teaspoon maple syrup

2 cups almond milk, unsweetened

Directions: Place all the ingredients in the order in a food processor or blender and then pulse for 2 to 3 minutes at high speed until smooth. Pour the smoothie into two glasses and then serve. Nutrition:

Calories: 324 Cal

Fat: 5 g

Carbs: 75.1 g

Protein: 7.2 g

Fiber: 11.3 g

Strawberry and Chocolate Milkshake

Preparation time: 5 minutes

Cooking time: 0 minute

Servings: 2

Ingredients:

2 cups frozen strawberries

3 tablespoons cocoa powder

1 scoop protein powder

2 tablespoons maple syrup

1 teaspoon vanilla extract, unsweetened

2 cups almond milk, unsweetened

Directions:

Place all the ingredients in the order in a food processor or blender and then pulse for 2 to 3 minutes at high speed until smooth.

Pour the smoothie into two glasses and then serve.

Nutrition:

Calories: 199 Cal

Fat: 4.1 g

Carbs: 40.5 g

Protein: 3.7 g

Fiber: 5.5 g

Banana and Protein Smoothie

Preparation time: 5 minutes

Cooking time: 0 minute

Servings: 2

Ingredients:

2/3 cup frozen pineapple chunk

10 frozen strawberries

2 frozen bananas

2 scoops protein powder

2 teaspoons cocoa powder

2 tablespoons maple syrup

2 teaspoons vanilla extract, unsweetened

2 cups almond milk, unsweetened

Directions

Place all the ingredients in the order in a food processor or blender and then pulse for 2 to 3 minutes at high speed until smooth.

Pour the smoothie into two glasses and then serve.

Nutrition:

Calories: 272 Cal

Fat: 3.8 g

Carbs: 59.4 g

Protein: 4.3 g

Fiber: 7.1 g

Mango, Pineapple and Banana Smoothie

Preparation time: 5 minutes

Cooking time: 0 minute

Servings: 2

Ingredients:

2 cups pineapple chunks

2 frozen bananas

2 medium mangoes, destoned, cut into chunks

1 cup almond milk, unsweetened

Chia seeds as needed for garnishing

Directions:

Place all the ingredients in the order in a food processor or blender and then pulse for 2 to 3 minutes at high speed until smooth.

Pour the smoothie into two glasses and then serve.

Nutrition:

Calories: 287 Cal

Fat: 1.2 g

Carbs: 73.3 g

Protein: 3.5 g

Fiber: 8 g

Blueberry and Banana Smoothie

Preparation time: 5 minutes

Cooking time: 0 minute

Servings: 2

Ingredients:

2 frozen bananas

2 cups frozen blueberries

2 cups almond milk, unsweetened

1/2 teaspoon or so cinnamon

dash of vanilla extract

Directions: Place all the ingredients in the order in a food processor or blender and then pulse for 2 to 3 minutes at high speed until smooth. Pour the smoothie into two glasses and then serve. Nutrition:

Calories: 244 Cal

Fat: 3.8 g

Carbs: 51.5 g

Protein: 4 g

Fiber: 7.3 g

'Sweet Tang' and Chia Smoothie

Preparation time: 5 minutes

Cooking time: 0 minute

Servings: 2

Ingredients:

4 large plums

2 tablespoon chia seeds

1/2 cup pineapple chunks

1/2 cup ice cubes

3/4 cup coconut water

Directions: Place all the ingredients in the order in a food processor or blender and then pulse for 2 to 3 minutes at high speed until smooth. Pour the smoothie into two glasses and then serve. Nutrition:

Calories: 406 Cal

Fat: 9.3 g

Carbs: 77.4 g

Protein: 6.3 g

Fiber: 13 g

Strawberry, Mango and Banana Smoothie

Preparation time: 5 minutes

Cooking time: 0 minute

Servings: 2

Ingredients:

1 medium frozen banana

1 cup of frozen strawberries

2 tablespoons ground chia seeds

1 cup chopped mango

2 tablespoons cashew butter

1 cup coconut milk, unsweetened

Directions:

Place all the ingredients in the order in a food processor or blender and then pulse for 2 to 3 minutes at high speed until smooth.

Pour the smoothie into two glasses and then serve.

Nutrition:

Calories: 299 Cal

Fat: 15 g

Carbs: 42 g

Protein: 5 g

Fiber: 8 g

Strawberry and Pineapple Smoothie

Preparation time: 5 minutes

Cooking time: 0 minute

Servings: 2

Ingredients:

2 cups frozen strawberries

2 tablespoons almond butter

2 cups chopped pineapple

1 ½ cup chilled almond milk, unsweetened

Directions: Place all the ingredients in the order in a food processor or blender and then pulse for 2 to 3 minutes at high speed until smooth. Pour the smoothie into two glasses and then serve.

Nutrition:

Calories: 255 Cal

Fat: 11 g

Carbs: 39 g

Protein: 6 g

Fiber: 8 g

Strawberry, Blueberry and Banana Smoothie

Preparation time: 5 minutes

Cooking time: 0 minute

Servings: 2

Ingredients:

1 tablespoon hulled hemp seeds

½ cup of frozen strawberries

1 small frozen banana

½ cup frozen blueberries

2 tablespoons cashew butter

¾ cup cashew milk, unsweetened

Directions:

Place all the ingredients in the order in a food processor or blender and then pulse for 2 to 3 minutes at high speed until smooth.

Pour the smoothie into two glasses and then serve.

Nutrition:

Calories: 334 Cal

Fat: 17 g

Carbs: 46 g

Protein: 7 g

Fiber: 7 g

Pineapple and Spinach Juice

Preparation time: 5 minutes

Cooking time: 0 minute

Servings: 2

Ingredients:

2 medium red apples, cored, peeled, chopped

3 cups spinach

½ of a medium pineapple, peeled

2 lemons, peeled

Directions: Process all the ingredients in the order in a juicer or blender and then strain it into two glasses. Serve straight away.

Nutrition:

Calories: 131 Cal

Fat: 0.5 g

Carbs: 34.5 g

Protein: 1.7 g

Fiber: 5 g

Green Lemonade

Preparation time: 5 minutes

Cooking time: 0 minute

Servings: 2

Ingredients:

10 large stalks of celery, chopped

2 medium green apples, cored, peeled, chopped

2 medium cucumbers, peeled, chopped

2 inches piece of ginger

10 stalks of kale, chopped

2 cups parsley

Directions:

Process all the ingredients in the order in a juicer or blender and then strain it into two glasses.

Serve straight away.

Nutrition:

Calories: 102.3 Cal

Fat: 1.1 g

Carbs: 26.2 g

Protein: 4.7 g

Fiber: 8.5 g

Sweet and Sour Juice

Preparation time: 5 minutes

Cooking time: 0 minute

Servings: 2

Ingredients:

2 medium apples, cored, peeled, chopped

2 large cucumbers, peeled

4 cups chopped grapefruit

1 cup mint

Directions: Process all the ingredients in the order in a juicer or blender and then strain it into two glasses.

Serve straight away.

Nutrition:

Calories: 90 Cal

Fat: 0 g

Carbs: 23 g

Protein: 0 g

Fiber: 9 g

Apple, Carrot, Celery and Kale Juice

Preparation time: 5 minutes

Cooking time: 0 minute

Servings: 2

Ingredients:

5 curly kale

2 green apples, cored, peeled, chopped

2 large stalks celery

4 large carrots, cored, peeled, chopped

Directions:

Process all the ingredients in the order in a juicer or blender and then strain it into two glasses. Serve straight away.

Nutrition:

Calories: 183 Cal

Fat: 2.5 g

Carbs: 46 g

Protein: 13 g

Fiber: 3 g

Banana Milk

Preparation time: 5 minutes

Cooking time: 0 minute

Servings: 2

Ingredients:

2 dates

2 medium bananas, peeled

1 teaspoon vanilla extract, unsweetened

1/2 cup ice

2 cups of water

Directions: Place all the ingredients in the order in a food processor or blender and then pulse for 2 to 3 minutes at high speed until smooth. Pour the smoothie into two glasses and then serve. Nutrition:

Calories: 79 Cal

Fat: 0 g

Carbs: 19.8 g

Protein: 0.8 g

Fiber: 6 g

Hazelnut and Chocolate Milk

Preparation time: 5 minutes

Cooking time: 0 minute

Servings: 2

Ingredients:

2 tablespoons cocoa powder

4 dates, pitted

1 cup hazelnuts

3 cups of water

Directions: Place all the ingredients in the order in a food processor or blender and then pulse for 2 to 3 minutes at high speed until smooth. Pour the smoothie into two glasses and then serve.

Nutrition:

Calories: 120 Cal

Fat: 5 g

Carbs: 19 g

Protein: 2 g

Fiber: 1 g

Chapter 18: Vegetable meats

Tofu Hoagie Rolls

Preparation time: 10 minutes

Cooking time: 20 minutes

Servings: 06

Ingredients:

½ cup vegetable broth

¼ cup hot sauce

1 tablespoon vegan butter

1 (16 ounce) package tofu, pressed and diced

4 cups cabbage, shredded

2 medium apples, grated

1 medium shallot, grated

6 tablespoons vegan mayonnaise

1 tablespoon apple cider vinegar

Salt and black pepper

4 6-inch hoagie rolls, toasted

Directions:

In a saucepan, combine broth with butter and hot sauce and bring to a boil.

Add tofu and reduce the heat to a simmer.

Cook for 10 minutes then remove from heat and let sit for 10 minutes to marinate.

Toss cabbage and rest of the ingredients in a salad bowl.

Prepare and set up a grill on medium heat.

Drain the tofu and grill for 5 minutes per side.

Lay out the toasted hoagie rolls and add grilled tofu to each hoagie

Add the cabbage mixture evenly between them then close it.

Serve.

Nutrition:

Calories 372

Total Fat 11.1 g

Saturated Fat 5.8 g

Cholesterol 610 mg

Sodium 749 mg

Total Carbs 16.9 g

Fiber 0.2 g

Sugar 0.2 g

Protein 13.5 g

Grilled Avocado with Tomatoes

Preparation time: 10 minutes

Cooking time: 15 minutes

Servings: 06

Ingredients:

3 avocados, halved and pitted

3 limes, wedged

1½ cup grape tomatoes

1 cup fresh corn

1 cup onion, chopped

3 serrano peppers

2 garlic cloves, peeled

¼ cup cilantro leaves, chopped

1 tablespoon olive oil

Salt and black pepper to taste

Directions:

Prepare and set a grill over medium heat.

Brush the avocado with oil and grill it for 5 minutes per side.

Meanwhile, toss the garlic, onion, corn, tomatoes, and pepper in a baking sheet.

At 550 degrees F, roast the vegetables for 5 minutes.

Toss the veggie mix and stir in salt, cilantro, and black pepper.

Mix well then fill the grilled avocadoes with the mixture.

Garnish with lime.

Serve.

Nutrition:

Calories 114

Total Fat 5.7 g

Saturated Fat 2.7 g

Cholesterol 75 mg

Sodium 94 mg

Total Carbs 31.4 g

Fiber 0.6 g

Sugar 15 g

Protein 4.1 g

Grilled Tofu with Chimichurri Sauce

Preparation time: 10 minutes

Cooking time: 12 minutes

Servings: 04

Ingredients:

2 tablespoons plus 1 teaspoon olive oil

1 teaspoon dried oregano

1 cup parsley leaves

½ cup cilantro leaves

2 Fresno peppers, seeded and chopped

2 tablespoons white wine vinegar

2 tablespoons water

1 tablespoon fresh lime juice

Salt and black pepper

1 cup couscous, cooked

1 teaspoon lime zest

¼ cup toasted pumpkin seeds

1 cup fresh spinach, chopped

1 (15.5 ounce) can kidney beans, rinsed and drained

1 (14 to 16 ounce) block tofu, diced

2 summer squashes, diced

3 spring onions, quartered

Directions:

In a saucepan, heat 2 tablespoons oil and add oregano over medium heat.

After 30 seconds add parsley, chili pepper, cilantro, lime juice, 2 tablespoons water, vinegar, salt and black pepper.

Mix well then blend in a blender.

Add the remaining oil, pumpkin seeds, beans and spinach and cook for 3 minutes.

Stir in couscous and adjust seasoning with salt and black pepper.

Prepare and set up a grill on medium heat.

Thread the tofu, squash, and onions on the skewer in an alternating pattern.

Grill these skewers for 4 minutes per side while basting with the green sauce.

Serve the skewers on top of the couscous with green sauce.

Enjoy.

Nutrition:

Calories 249

Total Fat 11.9 g

Saturated Fat 1.7 g

Cholesterol 78 mg

Sodium 79 mg

Total Carbs 41.8 g

Fiber 1.1 g

Sugar 0.3 g

Protein 1 g

Grilled Seitan with Creole Sauce

Preparation time: 10 minutes

Cooking time: 14 minutes

Servings: 04

Ingredients:

Grilled Seitan Kebabs:

4 cups seitan, diced

2 medium onions, diced into squares

8 bamboo skewers

1 can coconut milk

2½ tablespoons creole spice

2 tablespoons tomato paste

2 cloves of garlic

Creole Spice Mix:

2 tablespoons paprika

12 dried peri chili peppers

1 tablespoon salt

1 tablespoon freshly ground pepper

2 teaspoons dried thyme

2 teaspoons dried oregano

Directions:

Prepare the creole seasoning by blending all its ingredients and preserve in a sealable jar.

Thread seitan and onion on the bamboo skewers in an alternating pattern.

On a baking sheet, mix coconut milk with creole seasoning, tomato paste and garlic.

Soak the skewers in the milk marinade for 2 hours.

Prepare and set up a grill over medium heat.

Grill the skewers for 7 minutes per side.

Serve.

Nutrition:

Calories 213

Total Fat 14 g

Saturated Fat 8 g

Cholesterol 81 mg

Sodium 162 mg

Total Carbs 53 g

Fiber 0.7 g

Sugar 19 g

Protein 12 g

Mushroom Steaks

Preparation time: 10 minutes

Cooking time: 24 minutes

Servings: 04

Ingredients:

1 tablespoon vegan butter

½ cup vegetable broth

½ small yellow onion, diced

1 large garlic clove, minced

3 tablespoons balsamic vinegar

1 tablespoon mirin

½ tablespoon soy sauce

½ tablespoon tomato paste

1 teaspoon dried thyme

½ teaspoon dried basil

A dash of ground black pepper

2 large, whole portobello mushrooms

Directions:

Melt butter in a saucepan over medium heat and stir in half of the broth.

Bring to a simmer then add garlic and onion. Cook for 8 minutes.

Whisk the rest of the ingredients except the mushrooms in a bowl.

Add this mixture to the onion in the pan and mix well.

Bring this filling to a simmer then remove from the heat.

Clean the mushroom caps inside and out and divide the filling between the mushrooms.

Place the mushrooms on a baking sheet and top them with remaining sauce and broth.

Cover with foil then place it on a grill to smoke.

Cover the grill and broil for 16 minutes over indirect heat.

Serve warm.

Nutrition:

Calories 379

Total Fat 29.7 g

Saturated Fat 18.6 g

Cholesterol 141 mg

Sodium 193 mg

Total Carbs 23.7g

Fiber 0.9 g

Sugar 1.3 g

Protein 5.2 g

Zucchini Boats with Garlic Sauce

Preparation time: 10 minutes

Cooking time: 10 minutes

 Servings: 2

Ingredients:

1 zucchini

1 tbsp olive oil

Salt, to taste

Black pepper, to taste

Filling:

1 cup organic walnuts

2 tablespoons olive oil

½ teaspoon smoked paprika

½ teaspoon ground cumin

1 pinch salt

Sauce:

½ cup cashews

½ cup water

2 teaspoons olive oil

2 teaspoons lemon juice

1 clove garlic

⅛ teaspoon salt

Directions:

Cut the zucchini squash in half and scoop out some flesh from the center to make boats.

Rub the zucchini boats with oil, salt, and black pepper.

Prepare and set up a grill over medium heat.

Grill the boats for 5 minutes per side.

In a blender, add all the filling ingredients and blend them well.

Divide the filling between the zucchini boats.

Blend all of the sauce ingredients until it is lump free.

Pour the sauce over the zucchini boats.

Serve.

Nutrition:

Calories 268

Total Fat 6 g

Saturated Fat 1.2 g

Cholesterol 351 mg

Sodium 103 mg

Total Carbs 12.8 g

Fiber 9.2 g

Sugar 2.9 g

Protein 7.2 g

Grilled Eggplant with Pecan Butter Sauce

Preparation time: 10 minutes

Cooking time: 31 minutes

Servings: 02

Ingredients:

Marinated Eggplant:

1 eggplant, sliced

Salt to taste

4 tablespoons olive oil

¼ teaspoon smoked paprika

¼ teaspoon ground turmeric

Black Bean and Pecan Sauce:

⅓ cup vegetable broth

⅓ cup red wine

⅓ cup red wine vinegar

1 large shallot, chopped

1 teaspoon ground coriander

2 teaspoons minced cilantro

½ cup pecan pieces, toasted

2 roasted garlic cloves

4 small banana peppers, seeded, and diced

8 tablespoons butter

1 tablespoon chives, chopped

1 (15.5 ounce) can black beans, rinsed and drained

Salt and black pepper to taste

1 teaspoon fresh lime juice

Directions:

In a saucepan, add broth, wine, vinegar, shallots, coriander, cilantro and garlic.

Cook while stirring for 20 minutes on a simmer.

Meanwhile blend butter with chives, pepper, and pecans in a blender.

Add this mixture to the broth along with salt, lime juice, black pepper, and beans.

Mix well and cook for 5 minutes.

Rub the eggplant with salt and spices.

Prepare and set up the grill over medium heat.

Grill the eggplant slices for 6 minutes per side.

Serve the eggplant with prepared sauce.

Enjoy.

Nutrition:

Calories 201

Total Fat 32.2 g

Saturated Fat 2.4 g

Cholesterol 110 mg

Sodium 276 mg

Total Carbs 25 g

Fiber 0.9 g

Sugar 1.4 g

Protein 8.8 g

Sweet Potato Grilled Sandwich

Preparation time: 10 minutes

Cooking time: 12 minutes

Servings: 02

Ingredients:

1 small sweet potato, sliced

½ cup sweet bell peppers, sliced

1 cup canned black beans, roughly mashed

½ cup salsa

1 avocado, peeled and sliced

4 slices bread

1-2 tablespoons vegan butter

Directions:

Prepare and set up the grill over medium heat.

Grill the sweet potato slices for 5 minutes and the bell pepper slices for 3 minutes.

Spread each slice of bread liberally with butter.

On two of the bread slices, layer sweet potato slices, bell peppers, beans, salsa and avocado slices.

Place the other two slices of bread on top to make two sandwiches.

Cut them in half diagonally then grill the sandwiches for 1 minute per side.

Serve.

Nutrition:

Calories 219

Total Fat 19.7 g

Saturated Fat 18.6 g

Cholesterol 141 mg

Sodium 193 mg

Total Carbs 23.7 g

Fiber 0.2 g

Sugar 1.3 g

Protein 5.2 g

Grilled Eggplant

Preparation time: 10 minutes

Cooking time: 10 minutes

 Servings: 04

Ingredients:

2 tablespoons salt

1 cup water

3 medium eggplants, sliced

⅓ cup olive oil

Directions:

Mix water with salt in a bowl and soak eggplants for 10 minutes.

Drain the eggplant and leave them in a colander.

Pat them dry with a paper towel.

Prepare and set up the grill at medium heat.

Toss the eggplant slices in olive oil.

Grill them for 5 minutes per side.

Serve.

Nutrition:

Calories 248

Total Fat 15.7 g

Saturated Fat 2.7 g

Cholesterol 75 mg

Sodium 94 mg

Total Carbs 38.4 g

Fiber 0.3 g

Sugar 0.1 g

Protein 14.1 g

Grilled Portobello

Preparation time: 10 minutes

Cooking time: 8 minutes

Servings: 04

Ingredients:

4 portobello mushrooms

¼ cup soy sauce

¼ cup tomato sauce

2 tablespoons maple syrup

1 tablespoon molasses

2 tablespoons minced garlic

1 tablespoon onion powder

1 pinch salt and pepper

Directions:

Mix all the ingredients except mushrooms in a bowl.

Add mushrooms to this marinade and mix well to coat.

Cover and marinate for 1 hour.

Prepare and set up the grill at medium heat. Grease it with cooking spray.

Grill the mushroom for 4 minutes per side.

Serve.

Nutrition:

Calories 301

Total Fat 12.2 g

Saturated Fat 2.4 g

Cholesterol 110 mg

Sodium 276 mg

Total Carbs 12.5 g

Fiber 0.9 g

Sugar 1.4 g

Protein 8.8 g

Ginger Sweet Tofu

Preparation time: 10 minutes

Cooking time: 15 minutes

Servings: 04

Ingredients:

½ pound firm tofu, drained and diced

2 tablespoons peanut oil

1-inch piece ginger, sliced

⅓ pound bok choy, leaves separated

1 tablespoon shao sing rice wine

1 tablespoon rice vinegar

½ teaspoon dried chili flakes

Marinade:

1 tablespoon grated ginger

1 teaspoon dark soy sauce

2 tablespoons light soy sauce

1 tablespoon brown sugar

Directions:

Toss the tofu cubes with the marinade ingredients and marinate for 15 minutes.

In a wok, add half of the oil and ginger, then sauté for 30 secs.

Toss in bok choy and cook for 2 minutes.

Add a splash of water and steam for 2 minutes.

Transfer the bok choy to a bowl.

Add remaining oil and tofu to the pan then sauté for 10 minutes. Add the tofu to the bok choy.

Serve. Nutrition:

Calories 119

Total Fat 14 g

Saturated Fat 2 g

Cholesterol 65 mg

Sodium 269 mg

Total Carbs 19 g

Fiber 4 g

Sugar 6 g

Protein 5g

Singapore Tofu

Preparation time: 10 minutes

Cooking time: 8 minutes

Servings: 04

Ingredients:

3.5 ounces fine rice noodles, boiled

4 ounces firm tofu, boiled

2 tablespoons sunflower oil

3 spring onions, shredded

1 small piece of ginger, chopped

1 red pepper, thinly sliced

3.5 ounces snap peas

3.5 ounces beansprouts

1 teaspoon tikka masala paste

2 teaspoons reduced-salt soy sauce

1 tablespoon sweet chili sauce

Chopped coriander and lime

Lime wedges, to serve

Directions:

In a wok, add 1 tablespoon oil and the tofu then sauté for 5 minutes.

Transfer the sautéed tofu to a bowl.

Add more oil and the rest of the ingredients except noodles to the wok.

Stir fry for 3 minutes then add the tofu.

Toss well and then add noodles.

Mix and serve with lime wedges.

Nutrition:

Calories 231

Total Fat 20.1 g

Saturated Fat 2.4 g

Cholesterol 110 mg

Sodium 941 mg

Total Carbs 20.1 g

Fiber 0.9 g

Sugar 1.4 g

Protein 4.6 g

Wok Fried Broccoli

Preparation time: 10 minutes

Cooking time: 16 minutes

Servings: 02

Ingredients:

3 ounces whole, blanched peanuts

2 tablespoons olive oil

1 banana shallot, sliced

10 ounces broccoli, trimmed and cut into florets

¼ red pepper, julienned

½ yellow pepper, julienned

1 teaspoon soy sauce

Directions:

Toast peanuts on a baking sheet for 15 minutes at 350 degrees F.

In a wok, add oil and shallots and sauté for 10 minutes.

Toss in broccoli and peppers.

Stir fry for 3 minutes then add the rest of the ingredients.

Cook for 3 additional minutes and serve.

Nutrition:

Calories 361

Total Fat 16.3 g

Saturated Fat 4.9 g

Cholesterol 114 mg

Sodium 515 mg

Total Carbs 29.3 g

Fiber 0.1 g

Sugar 18.2 g

Protein 3.3 g

Broccoli & Brown Rice Satay

Preparation time: 10 minutes

Cooking time: 10 minutes

Servings: 4

Ingredients:

6 trimmed broccoli florets, halved

1-inch piece of ginger, shredded

2 garlic cloves, shredded

1 red onion, sliced

1 roasted red pepper, cut into cubes

2 teaspoons olive oil

1 teaspoon mild chili powder

1 tablespoon reduced salt soy sauce

1 tablespoon maple syrup

1 cup cooked brown rice

Directions:

Boil broccoli in water for 4 minutes then drain immediately.

In a pan add olive oil, ginger, onion, and garlic.

Stir fry for 2 minutes then add the rest of the ingredients.

Cook for 3 minutes then serve.

Nutrition:

Calories 205

Total Fat 22.7 g

Saturated Fat 6.1 g

Cholesterol 4 mg

Sodium 227 mg

Total Carbs 26.1 g

Fiber 1.4 g

Sugar 0.9 g

Protein 5.2 g

Sautéed Sesame Spinach

Preparation time: 1 hr. 10 minutes

Cooking time: 3 minutes

Servings: 04

Ingredients:

1 tablespoon toasted sesame oil

½ tablespoon soy sauce

½ teaspoon toasted sesame seeds, crushed

½ teaspoon rice vinegar

½ teaspoon golden caster sugar

1 garlic clove, grated

8 ounces spinach, stem ends trimmed

Directions:

Sauté spinach in a pan until it is wilted.

Whisk the sesame oil, garlic, sugar, vinegar, sesame seeds, soy sauce and black pepper together in a bowl.

Stir in spinach and mix well.

Cover and refrigerate for 1 hour.

Serve.

Nutrition:

Calories 201

Total Fat 8.9 g

Saturated Fat 4.5 g

Cholesterol 57 mg

Sodium 340 mg

Total Carbs 24.7 g

Fiber 1.2 g

Sugar 1.3 g

Protein 15.3 g

Chapter 19: Sandwiches and pizza

Fluffy Deep-Dish Pizza

Servings 6

Preparation time: 2 hours and 15 minutes

Ingredients:

12 inch of frozen whole-wheat pizza crust, thawed

1 medium-sized red bell pepper, cored and sliced

5-ounce of spinach leaves, chopped

1 small red onion, peeled and chopped

1 1/2 teaspoons of minced garlic

1/4 teaspoon of salt

1/2 teaspoon of red pepper flakes

1/2 teaspoon of dried thyme

1/4 cup of chopped basil, fresh

14-ounce of pizza sauce

1 cup of shredded vegan mozzarella

Directions:

Place a medium-sized non-stick skillet pan over an average heat, add the oil and let it heat.

Add the onion, garlic and let it cook for 5 minutes or until it gets soft.

Then add the red bell pepper and continue cooking for 4 minutes or until it becomes tender-crisp.

Add the spinach, salt, red pepper, thyme, basil and stir properly.

Cool off for 3 to 5 minutes or until the spinach leaves wilts, and then set it aside until it is called for.

Grease a 4-quarts slow cooker with a non-stick cooking spray and insert the pizza crust in it.

Press the dough into the bottom and spread 1 inch up along the sides.

Spread it with the pizza sauce, cover it with the spinach mixture and then garnish evenly with the cheese.

Sprinkle it with the red pepper flakes, basil leaves and cover it with the lid.

Plug in the slow cooker and let it cook for 1 1/2 hours to 2 hours at the low heat setting or until the crust turns golden brown and the cheese melts completely.

When done, transfer the pizza into the cutting board, let it rest for 10 minutes, then slice to serve.

Nutrition:

Calories:250 Cal, Carbohydrates:25g, Protein:5g, Fats:8g, Fiber:1g.

Incredible Artichoke and Olives Pizza

Servings 6

Preparation time: 1 hours and 50 minutes

Ingredients:

12 inch of frozen whole-wheat pizza crust, thawed

1 mushroom, sliced

1/2 cup of sliced char-grilled artichokes

1 small green bell pepper, cored and sliced

2 medium-sized tomatoes, sliced

2 tablespoons of sliced black olives

1/2 teaspoon of garlic powder

1 teaspoon of salt, divided

1/2 teaspoon of dried oregano

2 tablespoons of nutritional yeast

2-ounce cashews

2 teaspoons of lemon juice

3 tablespoon of olive oil, divided

8-ounce of tomato paste

4 fluid ounces of water

Directions:

Place the cashews in a food processor; add the garlic powder, 1/2 teaspoon of salt, yeast, 2 tablespoons of oil, lemon juice, and water.

Mash it until it gets smooth and creamy, but add some water if need be.

Grease a 4 to 6 quarts slow cooker with a non-stick cooking spray and insert the pizza crust into it.

Press the dough in bottom and spread the tomato paste on top of it.

Sprinkle it with garlic powder, oregano and top it with the prepared cashew mixture.

Spray it with the mushrooms, bell peppers, tomato, artichoke slices, olives and then with the remaining olive oil.

Sprinkle it with the oregano, the remaining salt and cover it with the lid.

Plug in the slow cooker and let it cook for 1 to 1 1/2 hours at the low heat setting or until the crust turns golden brown.

When done, transfer the pizza to the cutting board, let it rest for 10 minutes and slice to serve.

Nutrition:

Calories:212 Cal, Carbohydrates:39g, Protein:16g, Fats:5g, Fiber:5g.

Mushroom and Peppers Pizza

Servings 6

Preparation time: 2 hours

Ingredients:

12 inch of frozen whole-wheat pizza crust, thawed

1/2 cup of chopped red bell pepper

1/2 cup of chopped green bell pepper

1/2 cup of chopped orange bell pepper

3/4 cup of chopped button mushrooms

1 small red onion, peeled and chopped

1 teaspoon of garlic powder, divided

1 teaspoon of salt, divided

1/2 teaspoon of coconut sugar

1/2 teaspoon of red pepper flakes

1 teaspoon of dried basil, divided

1 1/2 teaspoon of dried oregano, divided

1 tablespoon of olive oil

6-ounce of tomato paste

1/2 cup of vegan Parmesan cheese

Directions:

Place a large non-stick skillet pan over an average heat, add the oil and let it heat.

Add the onion, bell peppers and cook for 10 minutes or until it gets soft and lightly charred. Then add the mushroom, cook it for 3 minutes and set the pan aside until it is needed.

Pour the tomato sauce, sugar, 1/2 teaspoon of the garlic powder, salt, basil, oregano, into a bowl and stir properly.

Grease a 4 to 6 quarts slow cooker with a non-stick cooking spray and insert the pizza crust into it.

Press the dough in bottom and spread the already prepared tomato sauce on top of it. Sprinkle it with the Parmesan cheese and top it with the cooked vegetable mixture.

Cover it with the lid, plug in the slow cooker and let it cook for 1 to 1 1/2 hours at the low heat setting or until the crust turns golden brown.

When done, transfer the pizza to a cutting board, sprinkle it with the remaining oregano, basil, then let it rest for 10 minutes and then slice to serve.

Nutrition:

Calories:188 Cal, Carbohydrates:27g, Protein:5g, Fats:5g, Fiber:3g.

Tangy Barbecue Tofu Pizza

Servings 6

Preparation time: 2 hours

Ingredients:

12 inch of frozen whole-wheat pizza crust, thawed

1 cup of tofu pieces

1 small red onion, peeled and sliced

1/4 cup of chopped cilantro

1 1/2 teaspoons of salt

3/4 teaspoon of ground black pepper

1 tablespoon of olive oil

1 cup of barbecue sauce

2 cups of vegan mozzarella

Directions:

Place a large non-stick skillet pan over an average heat, add 1 tablespoon of oil and let it heat.

Add the tofu pieces in a single layer sprinkle it with 1 teaspoon of salt, black pepper and cook for 5 to 7 minutes or until it gets crispy with a golden brown on all sides.

Transfer the tofu pieces into a bowl, add 1/2 cup of the barbecue sauce and toss it properly to coat.

Grease a 4 to 6 quarts slow cooker with a non-stick cooking spray and insert the pizza crust in it.

Press the dough into the bottom and spread the remaining 1/2 cup of the barbecue sauce.

Evenly garnish it with tofu pieces and onion slices.

Sprinkle it with the mozzarella cheese and cover it with the lid.

Plug in the slow cooker and let it cook for 1 to 1 1/2 hours at the low heat setting or until the crust turns golden brown.

When done, transfer the pizza into the cutting board, let it rest for 10 minutes and slice to serve.

Nutrition:

Calories:135 Cal, Carbohydrates:15g, Protein:6g, Fats:5g, Fiber:1g.

Tasty Tomato Garlic Mozzarella Pizza

Servings 6

Preparation time: 2 hours and 30 minutes

Ingredients:

12 inch of frozen whole-wheat pizza crust, thawed

3/4 teaspoon of tapioca flour

2 teaspoons of minced garlic

2 teaspoons of agar powder

1 teaspoon of cornstarch

1 teaspoon of salt, divided

1/2 teaspoon of red pepper flakes

1/2 teaspoon of dried basil

1/2 teaspoon of dried parsley

2 tablespoons of olive oil

1/4 teaspoon of lemon juice

3/4 teaspoon of apple cider vinegar

8 fluid ounce of coconut milk, unsweetened

Directions:

Start by preparing the mozzarella.

Place a small saucepan over a medium-low heat, pour in the milk and let it steam until it gets warm thoroughly.

With a whisker, pour in the agar powder and stir properly until it dissolves completely.

Switch the temperature to a low and pour in the salt, lemon juice, vinegar, and whisk them properly.

Mix the tapioca flour and cornstarch with 2 tablespoons of water before adding it to the milk mixture.

Whisk properly and transfer this mixture to a greased bowl.

Place the bowl in a refrigerator for 1 hour or until it is set.

Then grease a-4 to 6 quarts of the slow cooker with a non-stick cooking spray and insert pizza crust into it.

Press the dough into the bottom and brush the top with olive oil.

Spread the garlic and then cover it with the tomato slices.

Sprinkle it with salt, red pepper flakes, basil, and the oregano.

Cut the mozzarella cheese into coins and place them across the top of the pizza.

Cover it with the lid, plug in the slow cooker, let it cook for 1 to 1 1/2 hours at the low heat setting or until the crust turns golden brown and the cheese melts completely. When done, transfer the pizza to the cutting board, then let it rest for 5 minutes, and slice to serve.

Nutrition:

Calories:113 Cal, Carbohydrates:10g, Protein:7g, Fats:5g, Fiber:1g.

Delicious Chipotle Red Lentil Pizza

Servings 4

Preparation time: 1 hours and 45 minutes

Ingredients:

12 inch of frozen whole-wheat pizza crust, thawed

1/4 cup of red lentils, uncooked and rinsed

1/4 cup of chopped carrot

1 cups of chopped tomato

1 medium-sized tomatoes, sliced

2 green onions, sliced

1 chipotle chili pepper in adobo sauce. Chopped

1/2 cup of sliced olives

1/4 cup of chopped red onion

1/2 teaspoon of minced garlic

1/2 teaspoon of salt

1/4 teaspoon of ground black pepper

1/2 teaspoon of cayenne pepper

1/2 teaspoon of dried oregano

1 teaspoon of dried basil, divided

1 tablespoon of tomato paste

1 teaspoon of olive oil

1/2 teaspoon of apple cider vinegar

1 cup of water

1 cup crumbled almond ricotta cheese

Directions:

Place a medium-sized non-stick skillet pan over an average heat, add the oil and let it heat.

Add the onion, garlic and using the sauté button, heat it for 5 minutes or until the onions get soft.

Add the carrots, tomatoes, chipotle chile, oregano, 1/2 teaspoon of basil and stir properly.

Let it cook for 5 minutes before adding the lentils, salt, black pepper, cayenne pepper, vinegar, and water.

Stir properly, cook for 15 to 20 minutes or until the lentils get tender, thereafter, cover the pan partially with a lid.

In the meantime, grease a 4 to 6 quarts slow cooker with a non-stick cooking spray and insert pizza crust into it.

Press the dough into the bottom and spread the lentil mixture.

Spray it with the tomato slices, green onions, and olives.

Spread the cheese over the top and sprinkle it with the remaining 1/2 teaspoon of basil.

Cover it with the lid, plug in the slow cooker and let it cook for 1 hour or until the crust turns golden brown and allow the cheese to melt completely.

When done, transfer the pizza to the cutting board, then let it rest for 5 minutes, before slicing to serve.

Nutrition:

Calories:369 Cal, Carbohydrates:56g, Protein:5g, Fats:15g, Fiber:5g.

Chapter 20: Vegetable and vegan first courses.

Scrumptious Baked Potatoes

Servings 8

Preparation time: 8 hours and 10 minutes
Ingredients:

8 potatoes

Salt to taste for serving

Ground black pepper to taste for serving

Directions: Rinse potatoes until clean, wipe dry and then prick with a fork. Wrap each potato in an aluminum foil and place in a 6 to 8 quarts slow cooker. Cover with lid, and then plug in the slow cooker and let cook on low heat setting for 8 hours or until tender. When the cooking time is over, unwrap potatoes and prick with a fork to check if potatoes are tender or not. Sprinkle potatoes with salt, black pepper, and your favorite seasoning and serve.

Nutrition:

Calories:93 Cal, Carbohydrates:3g, Protein:3g, Fats:1g, Fiber:2g.

Fantastic Butternut Squash & Vegetables

Servings 6

Preparation time: 4 hours and 15 minutes

Ingredients:

1 1/2 cups of corn kernels

2 pounds of butternut squash

1 medium-sized green bell pepper

14 1/2 ounce of diced tomatoes

1/2 cup of chopped white onion

1/2 teaspoon of minced garlic

1/2 teaspoon of salt

1/4 teaspoon of ground black pepper

1 tablespoon and 2 teaspoons of tomato paste

1/2 cup of vegetable broth

Directions:

1— Peel, centralize the butternut squash and dice, and place it into a 6-quarts slow cooker.

2— Create a hole on the green bell pepper, then cut it into 1/2-inch pieces and add it to the slow cooker.

3— Add the remaining ingredients into the slow cooker except for tomato paste, stir properly and cover it with the lid.

4— Then plug in the slow cooker and let it cook on the low heat setting for 6 hours or until the vegetables get soft.

5— When 6 hours of the cooking time is done, remove 1/2 cup of the cooking liquid from the slow cooker.

6— Then pour the tomatoes mixture into this cooking liquid, stir properly and place it in the slow cooker.

7— Stir properly and continue cooking for 30 minutes or until the mixture becomes slightly thick.

8— Serve right away.

Nutrition:

Calories:134 Cal, Carbohydrates:23g, Protein:6g, Fats:2g, Fiber:4g.

Fabulous Glazed Carrots

Servings 5

Preparation time: 2 hours and 20 minutes

Ingredients:

1 pound of carrots

2 teaspoons of chopped cilantro

1/4 teaspoon of salt

1/4 cup of brown sugar

1/4 teaspoon of ground cinnamon

1/8 teaspoon of ground nutmeg

1 tablespoon of cornstarch

1 tablespoon of olive oil

2 tablespoons of water

1 large orange, juiced and zested

Directions:

1— Peel the carrots, rinse, cut it into 1/4-inch-thick rounds and place it in a 6 quarts slow cooker.

2— Add the salt, sugar, cinnamon, nutmeg, olive oil, orange zest, juice, and stir properly.

3— Cover it with the lid, then plug in the slow cooker and let it cook on the high heat setting for 2 hours or until the carrots become soft.

4— Stir properly the cornstarch and water until it blends well. Thereafter, add this mixture to the slow cooker.

5— Continue cooking for 10 minutes or until the sauce in the slow cooker gets slightly thick.

6— Sprinkle the cilantro over carrots and serve.

Nutrition:

Calories:160 Cal, Carbohydrates:40g, Protein:1g, Fats:0.3g, Fiber:2.3g.

Flavorful Sweet Potatoes with Apples

Servings 6

Preparation time: 5 hours

Ingredients:

3 medium-sized apples, peeled and cored

6 medium-sized sweet potatoes, peeled and cored

1/4 cup of pecans

1/4 teaspoon of ground cinnamon

1/4 teaspoon of ground nutmeg

2 tablespoons of vegan butter, melted

1/4 cup of maple syrup

Directions:

1— Cut the sweet potatoes and the apples into 1/2-inch slices.

2— Grease a 6-quarts slow cooker with a non-stick cooking spray and arrange the sweet potato slices in the bottom of the cooker.

3— Top it with the apple slices; sprinkle it with the cinnamon and nutmeg, before garnishing it with butter.

4— Cover it with the lid, plug in the slow cooker and let it cook on the low heat setting for 4 hours or until the sweet potatoes get soft.

5— When done, sprinkle it with pecan and continue cooking for another 30 minutes.

6— Serve right away.

Nutrition:

Calories:120 Cal, Carbohydrates:24g, Protein:1g, Fats:3g, Fiber:2g.

Fuss-Free Cabbage and Tomatoes Stew

Servings 6

Preparation time: 3 hours and 10 minutes

Ingredients:

1 medium-sized cabbage head, chopped

1 medium-sized white onion, peeled and sliced

28-ounce of stewed tomatoes

3/4 teaspoon of salt

1/4 teaspoon of ground black pepper

10-ounce of tomato soup

Directions:

1— Using a 6 quarts slow cooker, place all the ingredients and stir properly.

2— Cover it with the lid, plug in the slow cooker and let it cook at the high heat setting for 3 hours or until the vegetables gets soft.

3— Serve right away.

Nutrition:

Calories:103 Cal, Carbohydrates:17g, Protein:4g, Fats:2g, Fiber:4g.

Wonderful Glazed Root Vegetables

Servings 6

Preparation time: 4 hours and 20 minutes

Ingredients:

6 medium-sized carrots

4 medium-sized parsnips

1 pound of sweet potatoes

2 medium-sized red onions

1 teaspoon of salt

1/2 teaspoon of ground black pepper

5 teaspoons of chopped thyme

3 tablespoons of honey

1 tablespoon of apple cider vinegar

1 tablespoon of olive oil

Directions:

Peel the carrots, parsnip, sweet potatoes, onions, and cut it into 1-inch pieces.

Grease a 6 quarts slow cooker with a non-stick cooking spray, place the carrots, parsnip, onion in the bottom and then top it with the sweet potatoes.

Using a bowl whisk the salt, black pepper, 2 teaspoons of thyme, honey and oil properly.

Pour this mixture over on the vegetables and toss it to coat.

Cover it with the lid, then plug in the slow cooker and let it cook at the low heat setting for 4 hours or until the vegetables get tender.

When cooked, pour in the vinegar, stir, sprinkle it with the remaining thyme and serve.

Nutrition:

Calories:137 Cal, Carbohydrates:26g, Protein:2g, Fats:4g, Fiber:3g.

Super Aubergines

Servings 6

Preparation time: 8 hours and 15 minutes
Ingredients:

1 pound of eggplant

10-ounce of tomatoes, quartered

2-ounce of sun-dried tomatoes

1 small fennel bulb, sliced

1 medium-sized red onion, peeled and sliced

1/2 cup of chopped parsley

1/4 cup of chopped basil

1/4 cup of chopped chives

2 teaspoons of capers

1 teaspoon of minced garlic

1 1/2 teaspoon of salt

1 teaspoon of ground black pepper

1 teaspoon of coriander seeds

1 lemon, juiced

6 tablespoons of olive oil, divided

Directions:

Using a 6 quarts slow cooker, add 2 tablespoons of olive oil, top it with onions and garlic.

Remove the stem of the eggplant, cut it into 1/2-inch thick slices and brush 2 tablespoons oil on both sides of the eggplant slices.

Garnish the onion with the eggplant slices and cover it with tomato pieces, sun-dried tomatoes, and fennel slices.

Sprinkle it with salt, black pepper, and coriander seeds.

Cover it with the lid, then plug in the slow cooker and let it cook at the low heat setting for 6 to 8 hours or until vegetables gets tender.

While doing that, place the parsley, basil and chives in a food processor.

Add the remaining 2 tablespoons of olive oil along with the lemon juice, caper, and pulse it until it gets smooth.

When the vegetables are cooked, transfer it to a serving platter and drizzle it with the prepared herbs mixture.

Serve right away with crusty bread.

Nutrition:

Calories:62 Cal, Carbohydrates:12g, Protein:2g, Fats:2g, Fiber:4g.

Sweet and Spicy Red Thai Vegetable Curry

Servings 6

Preparation time: 4 hours and 45 minutes

Ingredients:

1/2 head cauliflower, chopped into florets

2 medium-sized sweet potatoes, peeled and cubed

1 cup of cooked green peas

8 ounces of chopped white mushrooms

1/4 cup of chopped cilantro, chopped

1 small white onion, sliced

1/2 teaspoon of salt

1 tablespoon of brown sugar

1/2 cup of toasted cashews

3 tablespoon of red curry paste

3 tablespoons of soy sauce

2 teaspoons of Sriracha sauce

14-ounce of coconut milk

Directions:

Grease a 6-quarts slow cooker with a non-stick cooking spray and add the cauliflower florets, sweet potatoes, and onion.

Using a bowl, stir properly the salt, sugar, red curry paste, soy sauce, Sriracha sauce and the coconut milk.

Pour this mixture on top of the vegetables in the slow cooker and toss it to coat properly.

Cover it with the lid, then plug in the slow cooker and let it cook at the low heat setting for 4 hours or until the vegetables get soft.

Then add the mushrooms, peas, to the slow cooker and continue cooking for 30 minutes.

Garnish it with cilantro and serve.

Nutrition:

Calories:141 Cal, Carbohydrates:13g, Protein:0g, Fats:9g, Fiber:3g.

Vibrant Minestrone

Servings 6

Preparation time: 6 hours and 25 minutes

Ingredients:

30 ounce of cooked cannellini beans

8 ounces of uncooked small pasta

12 thins of asparagus spears

3 carrots, peeled and sliced

6 ounces of chopped spinach

28 ounces of diced tomatoes

1 cup of cooked peas

1 medium-sized white onion, peeled and diced

1 1/2 teaspoon of minced garlic

1 teaspoon of salt

1/2 teaspoon of ground black pepper

3 cups of vegetable stock

3 cups of water

1/3 cup of grated parmesan cheese

Directions:

Grease a 6-quarts slow cooker with a non-stick cooking spray, add the beans, carrots, tomatoes, onion, garlic, vegetable stock and water.

Stir properly and cover it with the lid.

Then plug in the slow cooker and let it cook at the low heat setting for 4 hours or until the vegetables get soft.

While doing that cut the asparagus into three and when the vegetables are cooked add the asparagus to the slow cooker along with the peas, salt, black pepper, spinach, and pasta.

Continue cooking for 15 minutes.

Garnish it with cheese and serve.

Nutrition:

Calories:110 Cal, Carbohydrates:18g, Protein:5g, Fats:2g, Fiber:4g.

Awesome Spinach Artichoke Soup

Servings 6

Preparation time: 4 hours and 45 minutes

Ingredients:

15 ounces of cooked white beans

2 cups of frozen artichoke hearts, thawed

2 cups of spinach leaves

1 small red onion, peeled and chopped

1 teaspoon of minced garlic

1 teaspoon of salt

1/2 teaspoon of ground black pepper

2 teaspoons of dried basil

1 teaspoon of dried oregano

1/2 teaspoon of whole-grain mustard paste

2 1/2 tablespoons of nutritional yeast

1 1/2 teaspoons of white miso

4 tablespoons of lemon juice

16 fluid ounces of almond milk, unsweetened

3 cups of vegetable broth

1 cups of water

Directions:

Grease a 6-quarts slow cooker with a non-stick cooking spray, add the artichokes, spinach, onion, garlic, salt, black pepper, basil, and the oregano.

Pour in the vegetable broth and water, stir properly and cover it with the lid.

Then plug in the slow cooker and let it cook at the high heat setting for 4 hours or until the vegetables get soft.

While waiting for that, place the white beans in a food processor, add the yeast, miso, mustard, lemon juice and almond milk.

Mash until it gets smooth, and set it aside.

When the vegetables are cooked thoroughly, add the prepared bean mixture and continue cooking for 30 minutes at the high heat setting or until the soup gets slightly thick.

Garnish it with cheese and serve.

Nutrition:

Calories:200 Cal, Carbohydrates:13g, Protein:4g, Fats:12g, Fiber:2g.

Chapter 21: Dinner

Beans Curry

Preparation time: 10 minutes

Cooking time: 8 hours and 10 minutes

Servings: 5

Ingredients:

2 cups kidney beans, dried, soaked

1-inch of ginger, grated

1 ½ cup diced tomatoes

1 medium red onion, peeled, sliced

1 tablespoon tomato paste

1 teaspoon minced garlic

1 small bunch cilantro, chopped

½ teaspoon cumin powder

1 teaspoon salt

1 ½ teaspoon curry powder

2 tablespoons olive oil

2 tablespoons lemon juice

Directions:

Place onion in a food processor, add ginger and garlic, and pulse for 1 minute until blended.

Take a skillet pan, place it over medium heat, add oil and when hot, add the onion-garlic mixture, and cook for 5 minutes until softened and light brown. Then add tomatoes and tomato paste, stir in ½ teaspoon salt, cumin and curry powder and cook for 5 minutes until cooked.

Drain the soaked beans, add them to the slow cooker, add cooked tomato mixture, and remaining ingredients except for cilantro and lemon juice and stir until mixed. Switch on the slow cooker, then shut with lid and cook for 8 hours at high heat setting until tender. When done, transfer 1 cup of beans to the blender, process until creamy, then return it into the slow cooker and stir until mixed. Drizzle with lemon juice, top with cilantro, and serve. Nutrition:

Calories: 252 Cal

Fat: 6.5 g

Carbs: 38 g

Protein: 13 g

Fiber: 9.3 g

Pasta with Kidney Bean Sauce

Preparation time: 5 minutes

Cooking time: 15 minutes

Servings: 4

Ingredients:

12 ounces cooked kidney beans

7 ounces whole-wheat pasta, cooked

1 medium white onion, peeled, diced

1 cup arugula

2 tablespoons tomato paste

1 teaspoon minced garlic

½ teaspoon smoked paprika

1 teaspoon dried oregano

½ teaspoon cayenne pepper

1/3 teaspoon ground black pepper

2/3 teaspoon salt

2 tablespoons balsamic vinegar

Directions:

Take a large skillet pan, place it over medium-high heat, add onion and garlic, splash with some water and cook for 5 minutes.

Then add remaining ingredients, except for pasta and arugula, stir until mixed and cook for 10 minutes until thickened.

When done, mash with the fork, top with arugula and serve with pasta.

Serve straight away

Nutrition:

Calories: 236 Cal

Fat: 1.6 g

Carbs: 46 g

Protein: 12 g

Fiber: 12.3 g

Broccoli and Rice Stir Fry

Preparation time: 5 minutes

Cooking time: 10 minutes

Servings: 8

Ingredients:

16 ounces frozen broccoli florets, thawed

3 green onions, diced

½ teaspoon salt

¼ teaspoon ground black pepper

2 tablespoons soy sauce

1 tablespoon olive oil

1 ½ cups white rice, cooked

Directions:

Take a skillet pan, place it over medium heat, add broccoli, and cook for 5 minutes until tender-crisp.

Then add scallion and other ingredients, toss until well mixed and cook for 2 minutes until hot.

Serve straight away.

Nutrition:

Calories: 187 Cal

Fat: 3.4 g

Carbs: 33 g

Protein: 6.3 g

Fiber: 2.3 g

Lentil, Rice and Vegetable Bake

Preparation time: 10 minutes

Cooking time: 40 minutes

Servings: 6

Ingredients:

1/2 cup white rice, cooked

1 cup red lentils, cooked

1/3 cup chopped carrots

1 medium tomato, chopped

1 small onion, peeled, chopped

1/3 cup chopped zucchini

1/3 cup chopped celery

1 ½ teaspoon minced garlic

½ teaspoon ground black pepper

1 teaspoon dried basil

1 teaspoon ground cumin

1 teaspoon dried oregano

½ teaspoon salt

1 teaspoon olive oil

8 ounces tomato sauce

Directions:

Take a skillet pan, place it over medium heat, add oil and when hot, add onion and garlic, and cook for 5 minutes.

Then add remaining vegetables, season with salt, black pepper, and half of each cumin, oregano and basil and cook for 5 minutes until vegetables are tender.

Take a casserole dish, place lentils and rice in it, top with vegetables, spread with tomato sauce and sprinkle with remaining cumin, oregano, and basil, and bake for 30 minutes until bubbly.

Serve straight away.

Nutrition:

Calories: 187 Cal

Fat: 1.5 g

Carbs: 35.1 g

Protein: 9.7 g

Fiber: 8.1 g

Coconut Rice

Preparation time: 10 minutes

Cooking time: 25 minutes

Servings: 7

Ingredients:

2 1/2 cups white rice

1/8 teaspoon salt

40 ounces coconut milk, unsweetened

Directions: Take a large saucepan, place it over medium heat, add all the ingredients in it and stir until mixed. Bring the mixture to a boil, then switch heat to medium-low level and simmer rice for 25 minutes until tender and all the liquid is absorbed. Serve straight away.

Nutrition:

Calories: 535 Cal

Fat: 33.2 g

Carbs: 57 g

Protein: 8.1 g

Fiber: 2.1 g

Quinoa and Chickpeas Salad

Preparation time: 10 minutes

Cooking time: 0 minute

Servings: 4

Ingredients:

3/4 cup chopped broccoli

1/2 cup quinoa, cooked

15 ounces cooked chickpeas

½ teaspoon minced garlic

1/3 teaspoon ground black pepper

2/3 teaspoon salt

1 teaspoon dried tarragon

2 teaspoons mustard

1 tablespoon lemon juice

3 tablespoons olive oil

Directions:

Take a large bowl, place all the ingredients in it, and stir until well combined.

Serve straight away.

Nutrition:

Calories: 264 Cal

Fat: 12.3 g

Carbs: 32 g

Protein: 7.1 g

Fiber: 5.1 g

Brown Rice Pilaf

Preparation time: 5 minutes

Cooking time: 25 minutes

Servings: 4

Ingredients:

1 cup cooked chickpeas

3/4 cup brown rice, cooked

1/4 cup chopped cashews

2 cups sliced mushrooms

2 carrots, sliced

½ teaspoon minced garlic

1 1/2 cups chopped white onion

3 tablespoons vegan butter

½ teaspoon salt

¼ teaspoon ground black pepper

1/4 cup chopped parsley

Directions:

Take a large skillet pan, place it over medium heat, add butter and when it melts, add onions and cook them for 5 minutes until softened.

Then add carrots and garlic, cook for 5 minutes, add mushrooms, cook for 10 minutes until browned, add chickpeas and cook for another minute.

When done, remove the pan from heat, add nuts, parsley, salt and black pepper, toss until mixed, and garnish with parsley.

Serve straight away.

Nutrition:

Calories: 409 Cal

Fat: 17.1 g

Carbs: 54 g

Protein: 12.5 g

Fiber: 6.7 g

Barley and Mushrooms with Beans

Preparation time: 5 minutes

Cooking time: 15 minutes

Servings: 6

Ingredients:

1/2 cup uncooked barley

15.5 ounces white beans

1/2 cup chopped celery

3 cups sliced mushrooms

1 cup chopped white onion

1 teaspoon minced garlic

1 teaspoon olive oil

3 cups vegetable broth

Directions:

Take a saucepan, place it over medium heat, add oil and when hot, add vegetables and cook for 5 minutes until tender.

Pour in broth, stir in barley, bring the mixture to boil, and then simmer for 50 minutes until tender.

When done, add beans into the barley mixture, stir until mixed and continue cooking for 5 minutes until hot.

Serve straight away.

Nutrition:

Calories: 202 Cal

Fat: 2.1 g

Carbs: 39 g

Protein: 9.1 g

Fiber: 8.8 g

Vegan Curried Rice

Preparation time: 5 minutes

Cooking time: 25 minutes

Servings: 4

Ingredients:

1 cup white rice

1 tablespoon minced garlic

1 tablespoon ground curry powder

1/3 teaspoon ground black pepper

1 tablespoon red chili powder

1 tablespoon ground cumin

2 tablespoons olive oil

1 tablespoon soy sauce

1 cup vegetable broth

Directions:

Take a saucepan, place it over low heat, add oil and when hot, add garlic and cook for 3 minutes.

Then stir in all spices, cook for 1 minute until fragrant, pour in the broth, and switch heat to a high level.

Stir in soy sauce, bring the mixture to boil, add rice, stir until mixed, then switch heat to the low level and simmer for 20 minutes until rice is tender and all the liquid has absorbed.

Serve straight away.

Nutrition:

Calories: 262 Cal

Fat: 8 g

Carbs: 43 g

Protein: 5 g

Fiber: 2 g

Garlic and White Bean Soup

Cooking time: 10 minutes

Servings: 4

Ingredients:

45 ounces cooked cannellini beans

1/4 teaspoon dried thyme

2 teaspoons minced garlic

1/8 teaspoon crushed red pepper

1/2 teaspoon dried rosemary

1/8 teaspoon ground black pepper

2 tablespoons olive oil

4 cups vegetable broth

Directions:

Place one-third of white beans in a food processor, then pour in 2 cups broth and pulse for 2 minutes until smooth.

Place a pot over medium heat, add oil and when hot, add garlic and cook for 1 minute until fragrant.

Add pureed beans into the pan along with remaining beans, sprinkle with spices and herbs, pour in the broth, stir until combined, and bring the mixture to boil over medium-high heat.

Switch heat to medium-low level, simmer the beans for 15 minutes, and then mash them with a fork.

Taste the soup to adjust seasoning and then serve.

Nutrition:

Calories: 222 Cal

Fat: 7 g

Carbs: 13 g

Protein: 11.2 g

Fiber: 9.1 g

Coconut Curry Lentils

Preparation time: 10 minutes

Cooking time: 40 minutes

Servings: 4

Ingredients:

1 cup brown lentils

1 small white onion, peeled, chopped

1 teaspoon minced garlic

1 teaspoon grated ginger

3 cups baby spinach

1 tablespoon curry powder

2 tablespoons olive oil

13 ounces coconut milk, unsweetened

2 cups vegetable broth

For Serving:

4 cups cooked rice

1/4 cup chopped cilantro

Directions:

Place a large pot over medium heat, add oil and when hot, add ginger and garlic and cook for 1 minute until fragrant.

Add onion, cook for 5 minutes, stir in curry powder, cook for 1 minute until toasted, add lentils and pour in broth.

Switch heat to medium-high level, bring the mixture to a boil, then switch heat to the low level and simmer for 20 minutes until tender and all the liquid is absorbed.

Pour in milk, stir until combined, turn heat to medium level, and simmer for 10 minutes until thickened.

Then remove the pot from heat, stir in spinach, let it stand for 5 minutes until its leaves wilts and then top with cilantro.

Serve lentils with rice.

Nutrition:

Calories: 184 Cal

Fat: 3.7 g

Carbs: 30 g

Protein: 11.3 g

Fiber: 10.7 g

Tomato, Kale, and White Bean Skillet

Preparation time: 10 minutes

Cooking time: 10 minutes

Servings: 4

Ingredients:

30 ounces cooked cannellini beans

3.5 ounces sun-dried tomatoes, packed in oil, chopped

6 ounces kale, chopped

1 teaspoon minced garlic

1/4 teaspoon ground black pepper

1/4 teaspoon salt

1/2 tablespoon dried basil

1/8 teaspoon red pepper flakes

1 tablespoon apple cider vinegar

1 tablespoon olive oil

2 tablespoons oil from sun-dried tomatoes

Directions:

Prepare the dressing and for this, place basil, black pepper, salt, vinegar, and red pepper flakes in a small bowl, add oil from sun-dried tomatoes and whisk until combined.

Take a skillet pan, place it over medium heat, add olive oil and when hot, add garlic and cook for 1 minute until fragrant.

Add kale, splash with some water and cook for 3 minutes until kale leaves have wilted.

Add tomatoes and beans, stir well and cook for 3 minutes until heated.

Remove pan from heat, drizzle with the prepared dressing, toss until mixed and serve.

Nutrition:

Calories: 264 Cal

Fat: 12 g

Carbs: 38 g

Protein: 9 g

Fiber: 13 g

Chard Wraps with Millet

Preparation time: 25 minutes

Cooking time: 0 minute

Servings: 4

Ingredients:

1 carrot, cut into ribbons

1/2 cup millet, cooked

1/2 of a large cucumber, cut into ribbons

1/2 cup chickpeas, cooked

1 cup sliced cabbage

1/3 cup hummus

Mint leaves as needed for topping

Hemp seeds as needed for topping

1 bunch of Swiss rainbow chard

Directions:

Spread hummus on one side of chard, place some of millet, vegetables, and chickpeas on it, sprinkle with some mint leaves and hemp seeds and wrap it like a burrito.

Serve straight away.

Nutrition:

Calories: 152 Cal

Fat: 4.5 g

Carbs: 25 g

Protein: 3.5 g

Fiber: 2.4 g

Quinoa Meatballs

Preparation time: 10 minutes

Cooking time: 35 minutes

Servings: 4

Ingredients:

1 cup quinoa, cooked

1 tablespoon flax meal

1 cup diced white onion

1 ½ teaspoon minced garlic

1/2 teaspoon salt

1 teaspoon dried oregano

1 teaspoon lemon zest

1 teaspoon paprika

1 teaspoon dried basil

3 tablespoons water

2 tablespoons olive oil

1 cup grated vegan mozzarella cheese

Marinara sauce as needed for serving

Directions:

Place flax meal in a bowl, stir in water and set aside until required.

Take a large skillet pan, place it over medium heat, add 1 tablespoon oil and when hot, add onion and cook for 2 minutes.

Stir in all the spices and herbs, then stir in quinoa until combined and cook for 2 minutes.

Transfer quinoa mixture in a bowl, add flax meal mixture, lemon zest, and cheese, stir until well mixed and then shape the mixture into twelve 1 ½ inch balls.

Arrange balls on a baking sheet lined with parchment paper, refrigerate the balls for 30 minutes and then bake for 20 minutes at 400 degrees F. Serve balls with marinara sauce.

Nutrition:

Calories: 100 Cal

Fat: 100 g

Carbs: 100 g

Protein: 100 g

Fiber: 100 g

Stuffed Peppers with Kidney Beans

Preparation time: 5 minutes

Cooking time: 35 minutes

Servings: 4

Ingredients:

3.5 ounces cooked kidney beans

1 big tomato, diced

3.5 ounces sweet corn, canned

2 medium bell peppers, deseeded, halved

½ of medium red onion, peeled, diced

1 teaspoon garlic powder

1/3 teaspoon ground black pepper

2/3 teaspoon salt

½ teaspoon dried basil

3 teaspoons parsley

½ teaspoon dried thyme

3 tablespoons cashew

1 teaspoon olive oil

Directions:

Switch on the oven, then set it to 400 degrees F and let it preheat.

Take a large skillet pan, place it over medium heat, add oil and when hot, add onion and cook for 2 minutes until translucent.

Add beans, tomatoes, and corn, stir in garlic and cashews and cook for 5 minutes.

Stir in salt, black pepper, parsley, basil, and thyme, remove the pan from heat and evenly divide the mixture between bell peppers.

Bake the peppers for 25 minutes until tender, then top with parsley and serve.

Nutrition:

Calories: 139 Cal

Fat: 1.6 g

Carbs: 18 g

Protein: 5.1 g

Fiber: 3.3 g

Chapter 22: Desserts and snacks

Ginger-Spice Brownies

Preparation time 5 minutes

cook time: 35 minutes

Servings: 12 brownies

Ingredients:

1¾ cups whole-grain flour

1 teaspoon baking powder

1 teaspoon baking soda

½ teaspoon salt

1 tablespoon ground ginger

½ teaspoon ground cinnamon

½ teaspoon ground allspice

3 tablespoons unsweetened cocoa powder

½ cup vegan semisweet chocolate chips

½ cup chopped walnuts

1/4 cup canola oil

1/2 cup dark molasses

1/2 cup water

1/3 cup light brown sugar

2 teaspoons grated fresh ginger

Directions:

Preheat the oven to 350°F. Grease an 8-inch square baking pan and set aside. In a large bowl, combine the flour, baking powder, baking soda, salt, ground ginger, cinnamon, allspice, and cocoa. Stir in the chocolate chips and walnuts and set aside.

In medium bowl, combine the oil, molasses, water, sugar, and fresh ginger and mix well.

Pour the wet Ingredients into the dry Ingredients and mix well.

Scrape the dough into the prepared baking pan. The dough will be sticky, so wet your hands to press it evenly into the pan. Bake until a toothpick inserted in the center comes out clean, 30 to 35 minutes. Cool on a wire rack 30 minutes before cutting. Store in an airtight container.

Nutrition:

Calories: 258 Cal

Fat: 17 g

Carbs: 12 g

Protein: 14 g

Fiber: 2 g

Hummus without Oil

Servings: 6

Preparation Time: 5 minutes

Ingredients:

2 tablespoons of lemon juice

1 15-ounce can of chickpeas

2 tablespoons of tahini

1-2 freshly chopped/minced garlic cloves Red pepper hummus

2 tablespoons of almond milk pepper

Directions: Rinse the chickpeas and put them in a high-speed blender with garlic. Blend them until they break into fine pieces. Add the other ingredients and blend everything until you have a smooth paste. Add some water if you want a less thick consistency.Your homemade hummus dip is ready to be served with eatables!

Nutrition:

Fat – 3 g

Carbohydrates – 35 g

Protein – 11 g

Tempting Quinoa Tabbouleh

Servings: 6

Preparation Time: 10 minutes
Cooking Time: 10 minutes

Ingredients:

1 cup of well-rinsed quinoa

1 finely minced garlic clove

½ teaspoon of kosher salt

½ cup of extra virgin olive oil 2 tablespoons of fresh lemon juice Freshly ground black pepper

2 Persian cucumbers, cut into ¼-inch pieces 2 thinly sliced scallions

1 pint of halved cherry tomatoes ½ cup of chopped fresh mint

2/3 cup of chopped parsley

Directions:

Put a medium saucepan on high heat and boil the quinoa mixed with salt in 1 ¼ cups of water. Decrease the heat to medium-low, cover the pot, and simmer everything until the quinoa is tender. The entire process will take 10 minutes.

Remove the quinoa from heat and allow it to stand for 5 minutes. Fluff it with a fork.

In a small bowl, whisk the garlic with the lemon juice. Add the olive oil gradually. Mix the salt and pepper to taste.

On a baking sheet, spread the quinoa and allow it to cool. Shift it to a large bowl and mix ¼ of the dressing.

Add the tomatoes, scallions, herbs, and cucumber. Give them a good toss and season everything with pepper and salt. Add the remaining dressing.

Nutrition:

Fat – 20 g

Carbohydrates – 25 g

Protein – 5 g

Quick Peanut Butter Bars

Serving Size: 10

Servings: 1

Preparation Time: 10 minutes

Ingredients:

20 soft-pitted Medjool dates

1 cup of raw almonds

1 ¼ cup of crushed pretzels

1/3 cup of natural peanut butter

Directions:

Put the almonds in a food processor and mix them until they are broken.

Add the peanut butter and the dates. Blend them until you have a thick dough

Crush the pretzels and put them in the processor. Pulse enough to mix them with the rest of the ingredients. You can also give them a good stir with a spoon.

Take a small, square pan and line it with parchment paper. Press the dough onto the pan, flattening it with your hands or a spoon.

Put it in the freezer for about 2 hours or in the fridge for about 4 hours.

Once it is fully set, cut it into bars. Store them and enjoy them when you are hungry. Just remember to store them in a sealed container.

Nutrition:

Calories: 343 per serving Fat – 23 g

Carbohydrates – 33 g

Protein – 5 g

Healthy Cauliflower Popcorn

Servings: 2 cups

Preparation Time: 10 minutes

Cooking Time: 12 hours

Ingredients:

2 heads of cauliflower

Spicy Sauce

½ cup of filtered water

½ teaspoon of turmeric

1 cup of dates

2-3 tablespoons of nutritional yeast ¼ cup of sun-dried tomatoes

2 tablespoons of raw tahini

1-2 teaspoons of cayenne pepper 2 teaspoons of onion powder

1 tablespoon of apple cider vinegar 2 teaspoons of garlic powder

Directions:

Chop the cauliflower into small pieces so that you can have crunchy popcorn.

Put all the ingredients for the spicy sauce in a blender and create a mixture with a smooth consistency.

Coat the cauliflower florets in the sauce. See that each piece is properly covered.

Put the spicy florets in a dehydrator tray.

Add some salt and your favorite herb if you want.

Dehydrate the cauliflower for 12 hours at 115°F. Keep dehydrating until it is crunchy.

Enjoy the cauliflower popcorn, which is a healthier alternative!

Nutrition:

Calories: 69 per serving Fat – 2.4 g

Carbohydrates – 6 g

Protein – 3.1 g

Hummus Made with Sweet Potato

Servings: 3-4 cups

Preparation Time: 15 minutes
Cooking Time: 55 minutes

Ingredients:

2 cups of cooked chickpeas

2 medium sweet potatoes

3 tablespoons of tahini

3 tablespoons of olive oil

3 freshly peeled garlic gloves Freshly squeezed lemon juice

Ground sea salt

¼ teaspoon of cumin

Zest from half a lemon

½ teaspoon of smoked paprika

1 ½ teaspoons of cayenne pepper

Directions:

Preheat the oven to 400°F. Put the sweet potatoes on the middle rack of the oven and bake them for about 45 minutes.

You can also bake the potatoes in a baking dish. You will know that they are ready when they become soft and squishy.

Allow the sweet potatoes to cool down. Blend all the other ingredients in a food processor.

After the sweet potatoes have sufficiently cooled down, use a knife to peel off the skin.

Add the sweet potatoes to a blender and blend well with the rest of the ingredients.

Once you have a potato mash, sprinkle some sesame seeds and cayenne pepper and serve it!

Nutrition:

Calories: 33.6 per serving Fat – 0.9 g

Carbohydrates – 5,6 g

Protein – 1 g

Crisp Balls Made with Peanut Butter

Servings: 16 balls

Preparation Time: 29 minutes

Ingredients:

¼ cup of wheat germ

½ cup of natural peanut butter 1/3 cup of rolled oats

¼ cup of unsweetened flaked coconut ¼ cup of whole quick oats

½ teaspoon of ground cinnamon ¼ cup of brown rice crisp cereal 1 tablespoon of maple syrup

¼ cup of apple cider vinegar

Directions:

In a bowl, mix all the ingredients apart from the rice cereal. Combine everything properly.

Create 16 balls out of the mixture. Each ball should be 1 inch in diameter.

In a shallow dish, add the rice cereal and roll each ball on the crispiest. See that the balls are properly coated.

Enjoy your no-bake crisp balls.

Store them in a refrigerator for later use.

Nutrition:

Calories: 79 per serving Fat – 4.8 g

Carbohydrates – 6.3 g

Protein – 3.5 g

Healthy Protein Bars

Servings: 12 balls

Preparation Time: 19 minutes

Ingredients:

1 large banana

1 cup of rolled oats

1 serving of vegan vanilla protein powder

Directions:

In a food processor, blend the protein powder and rolled oats.

Blend them for 1 minute until you have a semi-coarse mixture. The oats should be slightly chopped, but not powdered.

Add the banana and form a pliable and coarse dough.

Shape into either balls or small bars and store them in a container.

Eat one and store the rest in an airtight container in the refrigerator!

Nutrition:

Calories: 47 per serving

Fat – 0.7 g

Carbohydrates – 8 g

Protein – 2.7 g

Zesty Orange-Cranberry Energy Bites

Preparation time 10 minutes

Servings: 12 bites

Ingredients:

2 tablespoons almond butter, or cashew or sunflower seed butter

2 tablespoons maple syrup, or brown rice syrup

¾ cup cooked quinoa

¼ cup sesame seeds, toasted

1 tablespoon chia seeds

½ teaspoon almond extract, or vanilla extract

Zest of 1 orange

1 tablespoon dried cranberries

¼ cup ground almonds

Directions:

Preparing the ingredients.

In a medium bowl, mix together the nut or seed butter and syrup until smooth and creamy. Stir in the rest of the ingredients, and mix to make sure the consistency is holding together in a ball. Form the mix into 12 balls.

Place them on a baking sheet lined with parchment or waxed paper and put in the fridge to set for about 15 minutes.

If your balls aren't holding together, it's likely because of the moisture content of your cooked quinoa. Add more nut or seed butter mixed with syrup until it all sticks together.

Per serving (1 bite) calories: 109; total fat: 7g; carbs: 11g; fiber: 3g; protein: 3g

Chocolate and walnut farfalle

Preparation time 10 minutes

cook time: 0 minutes

Servings: 4 servings

Ingredients:

½ cup chopped toasted walnuts

¼ cup vegan semisweet chocolate pieces

8 ounces farfalle

3 tablespoons vegan margarine

¼ cup light brown sugar

Directions:

In a food processor or blender, grind the walnuts and chocolate pieces until crumbly. Do not over process. Set aside.

In a pot of boiling salted water, cook the farfalle, stirring occasionally, until al dente, about 8 minutes. Drain well and return to the pot.

Add the margarine and sugar and toss to combine and melt the margarine.

Transfer the noodle mixture to a serving

Nutrition:

Calories: 258 Cal

Fat: 17 g

Carbs: 12 g

Protein: 14 g

Fiber: 2 g

Almond-date energy bites

Preparation time 5 minutes

Servings: 24 bites

Ingredients:

1 cup dates, pitted

1 cup unsweetened shredded coconut

¼ cup chia seeds

¾ cup ground almonds

¼ cup cocoa nibs, or nondairy chocolate chips

Directions:

Preparing the ingredients.

Purée everything in a food processor until crumbly and sticking together, pushing down the sides whenever necessary to keep it blending. If you don't have a food processor, you can mash soft medjool dates. But if you're using harder baking dates, you'll have to soak them and then try to purée them in a blender.

Form the mix into 24 balls and place them on a baking sheet lined with parchment or waxed paper. Put in the fridge to set for about 15 minutes. Use the softest dates you can find. Medjool dates are the best for this purpose. The hard dates you see in the baking aisle of your supermarket are going to take a long time to blend up. If you use those, try soaking them in water for at least an hour before you start, and then draining.

Per serving (1 bite) calories: 152; total fat: 11g; carbs: 13g; fiber: 5g; protein: 3g

Black sesame wonton chips

Preparation time 5 minutes

cook time: 5 minutes

Servings: 24 chips

Ingredients:

12 vegan wonton wrappers

Toasted sesame oil

1⁄3 cup black sesame seeds

Salt

Directions:

Preheat the oven to 450°f. Lightly oil a baking sheet and set aside. Cut the wonton wrappers in half crosswise, brush them with sesame oil, and arrange them in a single layer on the prepared baking sheet.

Sprinkle wonton wrappers with the sesame seeds and salt to taste, and bake until crisp and golden brown, 5 to 7 minutes.

Cool completely before serving. These are best eaten on the day they are made but, once cooled, they can be covered and stored at room temperature for 1 to 2 days.

Nutrition:

Calories: 258 Cal

Fat: 17 g

Carbs: 12 g

Protein: 14 g

Fiber: 2 g

Kale chips

Preparation time 5 minutes

cook time: 25 minutes

Servings: 2

Ingredients:

1 large bunch kale

1 tablespoon extra-virgin olive oil

½ teaspoon chipotle powder

½ teaspoon smoked paprika

¼ teaspoon salt

Directions:

Preparing the ingredients.

Preheat the oven to 275°f.

Line a large baking sheet with parchment paper. In a large bowl, stem the kale and tear it into bite-size pieces. Add the olive oil, chipotle powder, smoked paprika, and salt.

Toss the kale with tongs or your hands, coating each piece well.

Spread the kale over the parchment paper in a single layer.

Bake for 25 minutes, turning halfway through, until crisp.

Cool for 10 to 15 minutes before dividing and storing in 2 airtight containers.

Per serving: calories: 144; fat: 7g; protein: 5g; carbohydrates: 18g; fiber: 3g; sugar: 0g; sodium: 363mg

Tempeh-pimiento cheese ball

Preparation time 5 minutes

cook time: 30 minutes

Servings: 8 servings

Ingredients:

8 ounces tempeh, cut into 1/2-inch pieces

1 (2-ounce) jar chopped pimientos, drained

1/4 cup nutritional yeast

1/4 cup vegan mayonnaise, homemade or store-bought

2 tablespoons soy sauce

3/4 cup chopped pecans

Directions:

In a medium saucepan of simmering water, cook the tempeh for 30 minutes. Set aside to cool. In a food processor, combine the cooled tempeh, pimientos, nutritional yeast, mayo, and soy sauce. Process until smooth.

Transfer the tempeh mixture to a bowl and refrigerate until firm and chilled, at least 2 hours or overnight.

In a dry skillet, toast the pecans over medium heat until lightly toasted, about 5 minutes. Set aside to cool.

Shape the tempeh mixture into a ball, and roll it in the pecans, pressing the nuts slightly into the tempeh mixture so they stick. Refrigerate for at least 1 hour before serving. If not using right away, cover and keep refrigerated until needed. Properly stored, it will keep for 2 to 3 days.

Nutrition:

Calories: 258 Cal

Fat: 17 g

Carbs: 12 g

Protein: 14 g

Fiber: 2 g

Garlic toast

Preparation time 5 minutes

cook time: 5 minutes

Servings: 1 slice

Ingredients:

1 teaspoon coconut oil, or olive oil

Pinch sea salt

1 to 2 teaspoons nutritional yeast

1 small garlic clove, pressed, or ¼ teaspoon garlic powder

1 slice whole-grain bread

Directions:

Preparing the ingredients.

In a small bowl, mix together the oil, salt, nutritional yeast, and garlic.

You can either toast the bread and then spread it with the seasoned oil, or brush the oil on the bread and put it in a toaster oven to bake for 5 minutes.

If you're using fresh garlic, it's best to spread it onto the bread and then bake it.

Per serving (1 slice) calories: 138; total fat: 6g; carbs: 16g; fiber: 4g; protein: 7g

Vietnamese-style lettuce rolls

Preparation time 15 minutes

cook time: 0 minutes

Servings: 4 servings

Ingredients:

2 green onions

2 tablespoons soy sauce

2 tablespoons rice vinegar

1 teaspoon sugar

1⁄8 teaspoon crushed red pepper

3 tablespoons water

3 ounces rice vermicelli

4 to 6 soft green leaf lettuce leaves

1 medium carrot, shredded

1⁄2 medium English cucumber, peeled, seeded, and cut lengthwise into 1⁄4-inch strips

1⁄2 medium red bell pepper, cut into 1⁄4-inch strips

1 cup loosely packed fresh cilantro or basil leaves

Directions:

Cut the green part off the green onions and cut them lengthwise into thin slices and set aside. Mince the white part of the green onions and transfer to a small bowl. Add the soy sauce, rice vinegar, sugar, crushed red pepper, and water. Stir to blend and set aside.

Soak the vermicelli in medium bowl of hot water until softened, about 1 minute. Drain the noodles well and cut them into 3-inch lengths. Set aside.

Place a lettuce leaf on a work surface and arrange a row of noodles in the center of the leaf, followed by a few strips of scallion greens, carrot, cucumber, bell pepper, and cilantro. Bring the bottom edge of the leaf over the filling and fold in the two short sides. Roll up gently but tightly. Place the roll seam side down on a serving platter. Repeat with

Remaining ingredients. Serve with the dipping sauce.

Nutrition:

Calories: 258 Cal

Fat: 17 g

Carbs: 12 g

Protein: 14 g

Fiber: 2 g

Green goddess hummus

Preparation time: 5 minutes

cooking time: 0 minute

Servings: 6

Ingredients:

¼ cup tahini

¼ cup lemon juice

2 tablespoons olive oil

½ cup chopped parsley

¼ cup chopped basil

3 tablespoons chopped chives

1 large clove of garlic, peeled, chopped

½ teaspoon salt

15-ounce cooked chickpeas

2 tablespoons water

Directions:

Place all the ingredients in the order in a food processor or blender and then pulse for 3 to 5 minutes at high speed until the thick mixture comes together.

Tip the hummus in a bowl and then serve.

Nutrition:

Calories: 110.4 cal

Fat: 6 g

Carbs: 11.5 g

Protein: 4.8 g

Fiber: 2.6 g

Garlic, Parmesan and White Bean Hummus

Preparation time: 5 minutes

Cooking time: 0 minute

Servings: 6

Ingredients:

4 cloves of garlic, peeled

12 ounces cooked white beans

1/8 teaspoon salt

½ lemon, zested

1 tablespoon lemon juice

1 tablespoon olive oil

3 tablespoon water

1/4 cup grated Parmesan cheese

Directions:

Place all the ingredients in the order in a food processor or blender and then pulse for 3 to 5 minutes at high speed until the thick mixture comes together.

Tip the hummus in a bowl and then serve.

Nutrition:

Calories: 90 Cal

Fat: 7 g

Carbs: 5 g

Protein: 2 g

Fiber: 1 g

Tomato Jam

Preparation time: 10 minutes

Cooking time: 20 minutes

Servings: 16

Ingredients:

2 pounds tomatoes

¼ teaspoon. ground black pepper

½ teaspoon. salt

¼ cup coconut sugar

½ teaspoon. white wine vinegar

¼ teaspoon. smoked paprika

Directions:

Place a large pot filled with water over medium heat, bring it to boil, then add tomatoes and boil for 1 minute.

Transfer tomatoes to a bowl containing chilled water, let them stand for 2 minutes, and then peel them by hand.

Cut the tomatoes, remove and discard seeds, then chop tomatoes and place them in a large pot.

Sprinkle sugar over coconut, stir until mixed and let it stand for 10 minutes.

Then place the pot over medium-high heat, cook for 15 minutes, then add remaining ingredients except for vinegar and cook for 10 minutes until thickened.

Remove pot from heat, stir in vinegar and serve.

Nutrition:

Calories: 17.6 Cal

Fat: 1.3 g

Carbs: 1.5 g

Protein: 0.2 g

Fiber: 0.3 g

Kale and Walnut Pesto

Preparation time: 5 minutes

Cooking time: 10 minutes

Servings: 4

Ingredients:

1/2 bunch kale, leaves chop

1/2 cup chopped walnuts

2 cloves of garlic, peeled

1/4 cup nutritional yeast

½ of lemon, juiced

1/4 cup olive oil

¼ teaspoon. ground black pepper

1/3 teaspoon. salt

Directions:

Place a large pot filled with water over medium heat, bring it to boil, then add kale and boil for 5 minutes until tender.

Drain kale, then transfer it in a blender, add remaining ingredients and then pulse for 5 minutes until smooth.

Serve straight away.

Nutrition:

Calories: 344 Cal

Fat: 29 g

Carbs: 16 g

Protein: 9 g

Fiber: 6 g

Buffalo Chicken Dip

Preparation time: 5 minutes

Cooking time: 15 minutes

Servings: 4

Ingredients:

2 cups cashews

2 teaspoons garlic powder

1 1/2 teaspoons salt

2 teaspoons onion powder

3 tablespoons lemon juice

1 cup buffalo sauce

1 cup of water

14-ounce artichoke hearts, packed in water, drained

Directions:

Switch on the oven, then set it to 375 degrees F and let it preheat.

Meanwhile, pour 3 cups of boiling water in a bowl, add cashews and let soak for 5 minutes.

Then drain the cashew, transfer them into the blender, pour in water, add lemon juice and all the seasoning and blend until smooth.

Add artichokes and buffalo sauce, process until chunky mixture comes together, and then transfer the dip to an ovenproof dish.

Bake for 20 minutes and then serve.

Nutrition:

Calories: 100 Cal

Fat: 100 g

Carbs: 100 g

Protein: 100 g

Fiber: 100 g

Barbecue Tahini Sauce

Preparation time: 5 minutes

Cooking time: 0 minute

Servings: 8

Ingredients:

6 tablespoons tahini

3/4 teaspoon garlic powder

1/8 teaspoon red chili powder

2 teaspoons maple syrup

1/4 teaspoon salt

3 teaspoons molasses

3 teaspoons apple cider vinegar

1/4 teaspoon liquid smoke

10 teaspoons tomato paste

1/2 cup water

Directions:

Place all the ingredients in the order in a food processor or blender and then pulse for 3 to 5 minutes at high speed until smooth.

Tip the sauce in a bowl and then serve.

Nutrition:

Calories: 86 Cal

Fat: 5 g

Carbs: 7 g

Protein: 2 g

Fiber: 0 g

Vegan Ranch Dressing

Preparation time: 5 minutes

Cooking time: 0 minute

Servings: 16

Ingredients:

1/4 teaspoon. ground black pepper

2 teaspoons. chopped parsley

1/2 teaspoon. garlic powder

1 tablespoon chopped dill

1/2 teaspoon. onion powder

1 cup vegan mayonnaise

1/2 cup soy milk, unsweetened

Directions:

Take a medium bowl, add all the ingredients in it and then whisk until combined.

Serve straight away

Nutrition:

Calories: 16 Cal

Fat: 9 g

Carbs: 0 g

Protein: 0 g

Fiber: 0 g

Chapter 23: 18-Day meal plan.

DAYS	BREAKFAST	LUNCH/DINNER	SNACKS/DESSERTS
1	Sweet Potato Toasts	Tofu Hoagie Rolls	Ginger-Spice Brownies
2	Tofu Scramble Tacos	Grilled Avocado with Tomatoes	Hummus without Oil
3	Almond Chia Pudding	Grilled Tofu with Chimichurri Sauce	Tempting Quinoa Tabbouleh
4	Breakfast Parfait Popsicles	Grilled Seitan with Creole Sauce	Quick Peanut Butter Bars
5	Strawberry Smoothie Bowl	Mushroom Steaks	Healthy Cauliflower Popcorn
6	Peanut Butter Granola	Zucchini Boats with Garlic Sauce	Hummus Made with Sweet Potato

7	Apple Chia Pudding	Grilled Eggplant with Pecan Butter Sauce	Crisp Balls Made with Peanut Butter
8	Pumpkin Spice Bites	Sweet Potato Grilled Sandwich	Healthy Protein Bars
9	Lemon Spelt Scones	Grilled Eggplant	Zesty Orange-Cranberry Energy Bites
10	Veggie Breakfast Scramble	Grilled Portobello	Chocolate and walnut farfalle
11	Mango strawberry smoothie	Ginger Sweet Tofu	almond-date energy bites
12	Honeydew kiwi cooler	Singapore Tofu	Black sesame wonton chips
13	Frosty cappuccino	Wok Fried Broccoli	Kale chips

14	Pumpkin Spice Frappuccino	Broccoli & Brown Rice Satay	Tempeh-pimiento cheese ball
15	Cookie Dough Milkshake	Sautéed Sesame Spinach	Garlic toast
16	Strawberry and Hemp Smoothie	Beans Curry	Vietnamese-style lettuce rolls
17	Blueberry, Hazelnut and Hemp Smoothie	Pasta with Kidney Bean Sauce	Green goddess hummus
18	Mango Lassi	Broccoli and Rice Stir Fry	Garlic, Parmesan and White Bean Hummus

Conclusion

If you want to live a healthier and happier life, take the first step towards good nutrition.

Start with a diet like plant-based diet program, which has been proven in scientific research to be beneficial to health, but at the same time, is not too strict and stringent.

Follow the recipes and techniques presented in this book to achieve the best results.

Good luck!

CPSIA information can be obtained
at www.ICGtesting.com
Printed in the USA
LVHW010221021120
670427LV00001BA/35